What You Need to Know About PERNICIOUS ANAEMIA & VITAMIN B12 DEFICIENCY

Lately I stood at the bridge
in the brown night
From afar came a song:
a golden drop, it swelled
across the trembling surface
Gondolas, lights, music –
Drunken it swam out into the gloom…
My soul, a stringed instrument,
touched by invisible hands
sang to itself in reply a gondola song,
and trembled with gaudy happiness.
– Was anyone listening?

Friedrich Nietzsche
Ecce Homo – Why I Am So Wise

What You Need to Know About PERNICIOUS ANAEMIA & VITAMIN B12 DEFICIENCY

Martyn Hooper

With a Foreword by Dr Chris Steel MBE

BOOKS

Hammersmith Health Books
London, UK

First published in 2015 by Hammersmith Health Books – an imprint
of Hammersmith Books Limited
14 Greville Street, London EC1N 8SB, UK
www.hammersmithbooks.co.uk

British Library Cataloguing in Publication Data: A CIP record of this
book is available from the British Library.

Print ISBN 978-1-78161-051-0
Ebook ISBN 978-1-78161-052-7

Commissioning editor: Georgina Bentliff
Designed and typeset: Julie Bennett, Bespoke Publishing Ltd
Index: Dr Laurence Errington
Production: Helen Whitehorn, Path Projects Ltd
Printed and bound: TJ International Ltd, Padstow, Cornwall, UK
Cover design: Nicola Witt

Contents

Acknowledgements

As with my previous books I have received a great deal of help and encouragement from many people who have been kind enough to read the individual chapters and offer advice and observations. My thanks go to:

- Petra Visser of the Stitchting B_{12} Tekort Group in the Netherlands for her advice and suggestions on the content

- Professor David Smith who has once again offered so much support and advice

- Dr John Warren for his suggestions and corrections regarding new developments

- Professor Rob Poole for his patience and cooperation during our interview about mental health issues and pernicious anaemia

- Professor Mark Pritchard for his excellent elucidation of stomach cancer and pernicious anaemia

- Dr Willemina Rietsema and Miss Taylor Morgan for spending so much time reading, correcting and commenting on the first two chapters

- Professor David Wraith for answering my questions and explaining what could potentially be a cure for pernicious anaemia

- Dr Fiona Porter, Dr Andrew McCaddon and Peter Hudson for conducting and reporting on the first ever survey of pernicious anaemia patients' experiences

- Professor Jo Martin for making me aware of the *Atlas of Variation in Diagnostic Procedures* compiled by her and her team at the Department of Health, and to Right Care for permission to reproduce four maps from it

- The volunteers at the Pernicious Anaemia Society for all of their encouragement, support and commitment for no financial gain

- The trustees of the Pernicious Anaemia Society for placing their faith in me and for their encouragement and patience

- The members of the Pernicious Anaemia Society for providing me with case studies for the book – unfortunately limited space means that only a few could be used

- Georgina Bentliff of Hammersmith Health Books for her patience and encouragement

- Dr Chris Steele who was kind enough to read the final manuscript and write the foreword even though demands upon his time are great

- And finally my wife Cheryl for putting up with the clutter of books, research papers and various works in progress for the past six months and for her patience and support.

All the above have helped ensure that the contents of this book are as accurate as possible. If I have missed anyone out, I apologise, as I do for any errors within these covers. Despite all of the help I have received, any errors or omissions that are to be found are entirely due to my own inadequacies, for which I take the full blame.

Foreword

During my 45 years as a GP, I have often felt uneasy about the way in which pernicious anaemia is diagnosed and treated. This uneasiness has troubled me when initially investigating patients who complain of tiredness. After a preliminary clinical examination of the patient, I would order a series of blood tests, especially for anaemia, and, like most doctors, if the lab report came back showing no abnormal results, I would reassure the patient that all was well – he or she did not have anaemia.

In fact, all might not be well, because there is something disturbing going on here – 'normal' blood results indicating no anaemia might be very wrong with regard to an anaemia caused by vitamin B_{12} deficiency – pernicious anaemia.

I have felt a similar uneasiness when an affected patient has presented saying that he or she is still feeling tired despite receiving regular B_{12} injections, either self-administered or by way of the practice nurse. This tiredness should not be there if a patient is receiving regular intramuscular injections, but many of these patients experience a return of their symptoms, including feeling tired and exhausted, well before their next injection is due.

I have found that even checking patients' B_{12} levels would produce laboratory results showing that levels are not low, but still within the 'normal' range. Nevertheless, some of these patients just give themselves their B_{12} shots earlier than recommended and, low and behold, their tiredness clears and they feel normal again.

My uneasiness prompted me to begin listening to the patients; I took action not from a printed lab report but from what they were telling me... I started to pay attention to the patient not the paper.

My uneasiness was confirmed and explained when I attended a lecture by Martyn Hooper. Martyn, though not a doctor, is an expert on pernicious anaemia – a patient expert. He has not only suffered from pernicious anaemia for many years, but ended up with the serious consequences of undiagnosed and untreated disease. Martyn is the founder and current Chairman of the Pernicious Anaemia Society, and a very active and campaigning individual, but it's his own story and experience that are outstanding and, frankly, very disturbing.

Like many patients with pernicious anaemia, his general symptoms were put down to advancing age and also, in his particular case, to an unrelated fall. His condition was undiagnosed for many years because he learned to live with his symptoms – the constant tiredness, the mood swings and the difficulty in thinking clearly. Finally, through the intervention of his sister, who is a nurse, his blood picture revealed that he had almost no B$_{12}$ in his blood.

Martyn's lecture concentrated on the unreliable tests used to determine the B$_{12}$ status in patients and confirmed my uneasiness and subsequent changed attitude to 'normal' blood results. Living with this undiagnosed B$_{12}$ deficiency anaemia in his body and not receiving any treatment had produced serious problems for Martyn – this condition and subsequent effects were indeed 'pernicious'! Hearing Martyn's talk was enlightening; he confirmed my suspicions that patients with what appears to be 'normal' blood results may not, in fact, be 'normal', and when he revealed the series of obstacles that lie in the way of patients getting an accurate diagnosis of their condition I was truly shocked.

The whole background to this story is eloquently described in this very readable book. Pernicious anaemia was first identified in the mid-1800s, then later treated with raw liver extract, which is a source of vitamin B_{12} and which could, if taken in large enough doses, rectify a deficiency even in those who are unable actively to absorb B_{12} from food, including patients with pernicious anaemia. Synthesis of B_{12} as an injectable treatment in the 1950s changed the management of this disorder and the lives of thousands of patients.

One would say that this disease has been conquered – it can't be cured, but it can be treated with lifelong regular B_{12} injections. Yet despite the huge advances made in this diagnostic and therapeutic story, there are, today, still serious problems in the way pernicious anaemia is diagnosed and treated. By being aware of these problems both patients and practitioners can arrive at better outcomes.

Every doctor should read this book. Most doctors will learn something from it.

'Dr Chris' Steele MBE
GP Manchester
Resident doctor, ITV's *This Morning*

About the author

Martyn Hooper founded the Pernicious Anaemia Society to provide a forum for sufferers from the condition, who have suffered from vitamin B_{12} deficiency for many years without a diagnosis (see Appendix 1, Martyn's Story, page 241). To write this book – a follow-on from his earlier *Pernicious Anaemia: the forgotten disease* and *Living with Pernicious Anaemia and Vitamin B_{12} Deficiency* – he has drawn again on the experience of the Society's 7000+ members, together with the results of extensive new research into the condition.

Introduction

This book began life as the intended second edition of my first book – *Pernicious Anaemia: the forgotten disease* (which is now, by the way, referred to by most people as simply *'the forgotten disease'*); but it soon became clear that in the two and a half years since it was first published so many developments had taken place that needed to be included in any second edition, that the new edition would bear little resemblance to the original publication.   And not only have there been significant developments relating to a wide range of issues surrounding pernicious anaemia, but also certain facts and falsehoods have come to light that are certain to be of interest to patients and their families and friends and I have included these often astonishing findings throughout the chapters.

This book is not, therefore, intended to replace *'the forgotten disease'* but is a complement to it and readers who haven't read the first book might want to do so in order to fully understand the nature of pernicious anaemia and the problems that patients face when confronting the disease and, at the same time, help keep poverty at bay in the Hooper household.

There have been four main developments that have led to this completely new appraisal of pernicious anaemia.

Assay tests questioned

Firstly, just a few weeks after *'the forgotten disease'* was published, two important papers were published in the highly respectable *New England Journal of Medicine* that revealed serious short-comings in the current assay (test) that is used to determine the vitamin B$_{12}$ status in the blood of patients. The first of these papers showed that the presence of intrinsic factor blocking antibodies in a patient's blood was responsible for indicating false high levels of vitamin B$_{12}$ that would lead clinicians to rule out any B$_{12}$ deficiency and consequently pernicious anaemia.[1] And just a few weeks later more doubt was cast on the validity of the (still) currently used test by another paper published in the same journal.[2] What the authors of this second paper had done was to take frozen blood samples provided by patients many years earlier and analyse these samples on a modern machine. When they had been analysed a decade or so before, using the old assay machines, the blood was shown to be deficient in B$_{12}$. The results from the modern machines missed between 22% and 35% of patients with low B$_{12}$ status – it gave false high readings in 22–35%.[i] That would mean that between 22% and 35% of patients whose B$_{12}$ status was investigated would be told that they had no B$_{12}$ deficiency whereas of course they would be lacking in the essential vitamin.

This is what the authors of the second paper conclude: 'the diagnostic failures with all three CBLAs[ii] suggest widespread CBLA malfunction', and they realise that these 'malfunctions' have been going on for over a decade: 'the reports of errors that began in 2000 suggest that the CBLA problem is also long-standing'.

So who was to blame for this malfunctioning? Well, the authors lay the blame flatly on the manufacturers of the machines who

---

i The researchers investigated three different machines manufactured by different manufacturers which is why there are variations in percentages.
ii CBLA stands for competitive binding luminescence assay – that's the name given to the modern test.

had tried to get around the problem by sending out brochures suggesting that other tests be carried out in an effort to correct any discrepancies: 'CBLA brochures that advise users to test for anti-intrinsic factor antibodies when they are uncertain about a normal cobalamin result ignore the higher priority of preventing the CBLA-specific malfunction in the first place.'

Finally the authors request that the manufacturers should stop messing around and solve the problem: 'Manufacturers, who have access to proprietary information, must instead transparently identify and permanently correct the defect or defects.' That is the academic equivalent of a damn good rollicking. There have been some developments relating to this which will be discussed later when we talk of the 'active B_{12} test'.

Pernicious Anaemia Society survey

The second major development was the publication of the results of the Pernicious Anaemia Society's survey of members' experiences in getting diagnosed and treated that was published in April 2014 in the *British Journal of Nursing*.[3] The survey was designed by Dr Fiona Porter, a GP working in Wales and who is herself a sufferer and a member of the Pernicious Anaemia Society. Members of the Society were invited to complete a questionnaire, either online or via a paper copy, over an 18-month period. When nearly 1,300 responses were gathered it was time to 'clean' the data and this was carried out by Mr Peter Hudson, a biochemist with an interest in statistical modelling. Once the data was 'clean' it then had to be written up in a format that would be acceptable to publishers. This was completed by Dr Andrew McCaddon, a GP from the north of Wales who has long had an interest in all things to do with vitamin B_{12}. The paper was then tweaked for individual journals that it would be sent to and, after five months perseverance and three rejections, the paper was finally accepted for publication by the *British Journal of Nursing*.[iii]

The findings of the paper were startling for three reasons. Firstly, it was the first time any study had taken place into the experiences of patients in getting diagnosed and treated for pernicious anaemia. And for the first time, therefore, the Society had firm evidence, based on its members' experiences, of the serious failings in the way in which pernicious anaemia in particular, and B$_{12}$ deficiency in general, is diagnosed and treated. Secondly, and again for the first time, here was a set of data that echoed the enormous amount of anecdotal evidence from various social media and internet sites which indicated that there really are serious problems with the way in which pernicious anaemia is diagnosed and treated. And finally, the paper was important because it showed how the failings of the current assays are impacting on the everyday lives of patients and leading to all manner of problems. I shall be continually quoting results of the survey throughout this book whenever I refer to 'the survey'.

New BCSH guidelines

The third substantial development has been the publication in June of 2014 of the new *Guidelines for the diagnosis and treatment of cobalamin and folate disorders'* by the British Committee for Standards in Haematology.[4] In May 2012, following the intervention by the then Minister for Health, Paul Burstow MP, Carrie-Anne Carr[iv] and I met with two senior figures in the UK's Department of Health. One was the immediate past Chairman of

---

iii One well-known British journal rejected it within two hours due to its being 'too big' an issue.
iv An active member of the Pernicious Anaemia Society.

the British Committee for Standards in Haematology (which is a committee of the British Society for Haematology) and the other the then National Clinical Director of Pathology. The meeting was scheduled to last no longer than 30 minutes and Carrie and I believed it would last no more than 15 minutes. We began to explain the problems our members faced in getting diagnosed and treated quickly and adequately. We began to off-load some of our problems. After an hour the fire alarm sounded and it was announced that a bomb scare evacuation drill was in progress as part of the preparations for the London Olympics. A fire warden popped his head into the meeting room and told us we were to evacuate the building immediately. One of the doctors informed him that the meeting was so important that nobody in the room would be taking part, and 'Anyway,' he said, pointing at me, 'he can't descend stairs and we can't use the lifts.' The fire warden shrugged his shoulders and closed the door and returned to the organised chaos that was taking place in the corridors. I think it was around one and a half hours later that the meeting ended, the final comment being, 'Obviously we have a lot to discuss.'

We still don't know for certain whether that intensive and productive meeting was the reason why the new guidelines were produced, but I believe it was. It was such a relief to be listened to by senior decision-makers in health matters. Anyway, 18 months later I was sent a draft copy of the new guidelines. I wasn't asked to comment on them, I was just sent a copy as a matter of courtesy. I replied to the authors that they were to be congratulated on such a comprehensive review – that's all I could comment on. I am a lay person with no scientific qualifications or background and it would be for others to comment on the exact content, although I did, of course, read the guidelines thoroughly. And I was both delighted and disappointed. For although the new guidelines address the problems with the current assay (as outlined above), they did nothing to address the problems patients have in getting treated according to their individual needs. My private appraisal was 'Good, could have done better.'

NHS Atlas of Variation in Diagnostic Services

The final development that has led to this book was the production in November 2013 of the 'NHS Atlas of Variation in Diagnostic Services'[5] which is just that – an atlas of England (no such animal exists for the rest of the UK and, as far as I can determine any other part of the world) that shows by geographic area what tests are ordered and how many tests are requested by medical professionals (some are not requested by GPs but by specialists and other clinicians) per 1,000 patient group – so it isn't based on just individual trusts or surgeries but per 1,000 patients. It is a remarkable book that must have taken an enormous effort to produce.

One interesting aspect of the *Atlas* is that it provides information about routine screening of patients. It has long been contended by patients' groups associated with pernicious anaemia and B_{12} deficiency that the population should be routinely screened to identify any deficiency. Indeed, it is difficult to argue against a screening programme for B_{12} considering how widespread it is. The *Atlas* addresses this problem and sets out the case against screening the population for B_{12} deficiency. We'll examine this in more detail later.

The challenge of understanding pernicious anaemia

For the past two years I have busied myself in the business of the Pernicious Anaemia Society which is, at the end of the day, a patient support group. As well as offering sympathy, advice and information to members of the Society and their families and friends I have been doing what all patient support groups do – raising awareness among doctors and other scientists of the problems with the diagnosis and treatment of pernicious anaemia. As a patient support group that is all we can do. Contrary to what some believe we cannot tell doctors what to do, nor can we insist that those with the relevant knowledge investigate the problems faced by members of the Society. All we can do is raise awareness of these problems and, using tact, diplomacy and sensitivity build relationships with health researchers and decision-makers. And that is what the Society has done which is why it is now a recognised and accepted agent of patients with pernicious anaemia.

What we, as a Society, cannot be seen to do is run around waving our hands in the air shouting 'it's so unfair' – that was the advice given to me by one of the most senior figures in the UK's Health Service; advice that made complete sense to me. All I can do, as Chairman of the Pernicious Anaemia Society, is raise awareness among scientists, healthcare providers and the general public that there is a need for pernicious anaemia to once again be the subject of investigation by those who are qualified and able to do so – and that's a difficult thing to do because pernicious anaemia as a topic for medical research was put to bed many decades ago.

I have a book, published in 1976, that gives a doctor's account of the history of pernicious anaemia and how this disease occupied some of the greatest minds in medicine for 150 years. The Preface demonstrates that pernicious anaemia was a serious disease and the subject of demanding and thorough research for decades until doctors and scientists became satisfied that they had mastered the disease by using replacement therapy injections of vitamin B_{12}. This is what the Preface says:

The story of pernicious anaemia is one of the great

dramas in the history of medicine. From the opening scenes in which pernicious anaemia was described by Combe in 1822 and Addison in 1849, to the 'thickening of the plot' with the clinical accounts of Biermer in 1872 and the morphological observations of Ehrlich in 1880, to the dénouement in the great empirical discovery of liver therapy by Minot and Murphy in 1926, and the final scenes culminating in the isolation and crystallization of vitamin B$_{12}$ from liver extracts by Rickes et al. and Smith in 1948, the elucidation of the molecular structure of vitamin B$_{12}$ by Hodgkin in 1956, and the total synthesis of vitamin B$_{12}$ by Woodward in 1972, the saga of pernicious anaemia remains one of the most compelling accounts in man's conquest and understanding of disease.[6]

During the 30 years up until 1956 six Nobel prizes were awarded to doctors and scientists for their work on pernicious anaemia and vitamin B$_{12}$. The production of artificial vitamin B$_{12}$ and its application to treat, if not to cure, pernicious anaemia meant that the attention of doctors was now directed towards other diseases and pernicious anaemia, once a subject right at the front of medical research and responsible for some of the greatest medical discoveries of all time slipped quietly off the medical radar and became buried at the bottom of a large pile of papers marked as 'solved'. And this is why it is so difficult to get scientists to revisit the disease. The vast majority of doctors believe that pernicious anaemia is now no longer inevitably fatal and as a consequence the disease is no longer pernicious because injections of vitamin B$_{12}$ will ensure that the patient lives a happy and normal life.

This isn't the case for a large number of patients who still struggle with everyday living because they still suffer from the symptoms of the disease to a greater or lesser extent. There is no reliable explanation of why this group of hapless patients still experience the worst aspects of the disease just as there is no scientific basis to explain why some patients need much more frequent replacement B_{12} injections than others. And it is because doctors think that pernicious anaemia is 'old hat' and not a serious contender for in-depth research programmes that the Pernicious Anaemia Society has struggled to get doctors to revisit the disease.

On the other hand, whilst pernicious anaemia is not the subject of serious research, vitamin B_{12} continues to fascinate a dedicated group of doctors and scientists who have been battling for many years to uncover the vitamin's inner secrets. Whilst pernicious anaemia is no longer the centre of attention that it once was to the scientific community, vitamin B_{12} continues to fascinate and intrigue a not insignificant number of researchers who are determined to unravel the mysteries of the vitamin.

Here's how one such researcher put it in 1988: 'To the stalwart little band of investigators of vitamin B_{12} – now more rationally termed cobalamin – there is comfort in knowing that the stream of important scientific problems will never end.'[7] And the author doesn't see the vitamin yielding up its secrets easily – 'If the past is any guide to the future, they will be difficult problems inciting tumult and controversy, and in the end they will yield broad biologic insights and many surprises.'

And this isn't an isolated case. Just a few years ago another team of researchers had this to say about B_{12}:

> Many of the early clinical studies recognized that vitamin B_{12} deficiency also caused a severe neuropathy leading to paralysis and death, while post mortem analysis demonstrated spinal cord demyelination. Vitamin B_{12} is still the subject of intense research and, in particular, its role in preventing these irreversible neurological lesions remains unclear.[8]

When you begin to dig around a little, this small but highly active community of clinicians and scientists begins to reveal itself. There are several conferences held every year in various locations across the globe where delegates present and receive papers published on a whole raft of issues that revolve around vitamin B$_{12}$ and folate. And whilst the vitamin seems reluctant to yield the innermost secrets of its persona there is a general trend towards understanding more about this essential component of life though the biochemistry involved is far beyond my understanding. Pernicious anaemia as a serious research subject may have been largely forgotten but vitamin B$_{12}$ remains the subject of intense scrutiny by an enthusiastic and committed band of scientists.

As the Founder and current Chairman of the Pernicious Anaemia Society I am in a unique position to understand how the disease impacts on patients' lives; but more than that I am fully aware that there remain fundamental questions about pernicious anaemia that need answering, not just to contribute to scientific knowledge but to eliminate the sometimes debilitating symptoms that a great many patients continue to experience after their B$_{12}$ deficiency has been corrected. Why is this so? Why do some patients need much more frequent replacement B$_{12}$ injections than others and in greater concentrations? Why does it take so long for some patients to receive a diagnosis? These are just some of the questions that are specific to pernicious anaemia that need to be addressed if all patients with pernicious anaemia are to lead a normal and active life after being diagnosed and treated as they did before their illness. The Pernicious Anaemia Society is constantly raising awareness of these questions and a list of the top 10 queries we are asked are listed in Appendix 7 (see page 267), with the answers that we currently give to enquirers. Hopefully, this book will go some way in bringing about a renewed interest in pernicious anaemia among medical and scientific professionals.

References

1 Yang D, Cook R. Spurious elevations of vitamin B_{12} in pernicious anaemia. *New England Journal of Medicine* 2012; 366;18:1742-1743.

2 Carmel R, Agrawal Y. Failures of cobalamin assays in pernicious anemia. *New England Journal of Medicine* 2012; 367;4:385-386.

3 Hooper M, Hudson P, Porter F, McCaddon A. Patients journeys; the diagnosis and treatment of pernicious anaemia. *British Journal of Nursing* 2014; 23;7:16-21.

4 Devalia V, Hamilton MS, Molloy A-M. Guidelines for the diagnosis and treatment of cobalamin and folate disorders. *British Journal of Haematology* 2014; 166(4):496–513.

5 Public Health England. *The NHS Atlas of Variation in Diagnostic Services*, RightCare NHS; 2013. http://www.rightcare.nhs.uk/index.php/atlas/diagnostics-the-nhs-atlas-of-variation-in-diagnostics-services/ (accessed 24 May 2015).

6 Kass L. *Pernicious Anemia*. Volume VII in the series Major Problems in Internal Medicine. Philadelphia: WB Saunders Company;1976.

7 Beck WS. Cobalamin and the nervous system. *New England Journal of Medicine* 1988; 318:1752–1754.

8 Scott JM, Molloy A-M. The discovery of vitamin B_{12}. *Annals of Nutrition and Metabolism* 2012; 61(3):239–45.

Chapter 1

Blood, anaemia, pernicious anaemia and vitamin B$_{12}$ deficiency

When I was eventually diagnosed as having pernicious anaemia, I took it upon myself to try to find out as much about the disease as I could and, before very long, I found myself wishing that I had paid more attention to my science teachers in secondary school as I struggled to grasp the very basics of biology and chemistry. Thankfully, due to the internet and the patience and enthusiasm of various members of the scientific community, I started to understand what had happened to me that had caused me to develop pernicious anaemia. It also became quite clear early on in my investigations that there was a great deal of confusion over the different types of anaemias and how pernicious anaemia differed from B$_{12}$ deficiency. In this chapter I will try to explain these differences, but that will require some knowledge of basic biochemistry and so it's fitting that we begin our journey by looking at the smallest of all living things – cells.

Cells

To even begin to understand the nature of blood and different anaemias we first have to grasp the basics of cellular biology. You, like me, are made up of cells, unless that is you are a robot and a literate one at that. Cells were first discovered by the English natural philosopher Robert Hooke in 1665, who named them cells after the Latin 'cella', meaning a small room like those inhabited by monks at the time. Cell theory is the basis of biology and states that all organisms are made up of cells. Cells are the most basic unit of life and you are composed of around 75 trillion of them. A cell is a very busy place that has been defined as a 'vast teeming metropolis' by the biochemist Guy Brown and 'a complex chemical refinery' by James Trefil, the physicist (see Figure 1.1). It is a refinery because it is home to some very complex chemical goings-on and a metropolis because it is full of activity and powered by electricity.

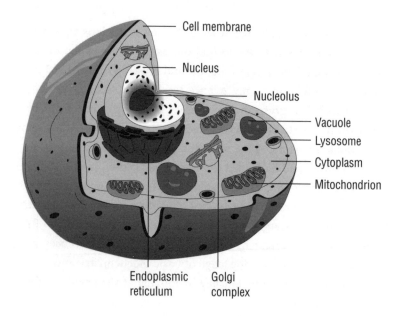

Figure 1.1 Anatomy of an animal cell

A cell is made up of millions of entities, including 'endosomes', 'ligands', 'lysosomes', 'peroxisomes' and proteins, and these carry out all manner of tasks, including extracting energy from food, carrying out repairs, getting rid of waste, sending messages and tackling intruders. While we needn't go into each of these entities in detail, one very important part of the cell is an organelle called a *mitochondrion*[i] which produces energy for the body – they (plural: *mitochondria*) are usually likened to the cell's battery pack, which provides the energy that allows cells to go about doing what they do – which allows you to live.

There are many different types of human cells but the one that is of greatest interest to us is one particular type – the red blood cell.

Blood

Saying that blood is a complicated substance is somewhat of an understatement – a bit like saying that the maiden voyage of the *Titanic* didn't go well. Blood is an extremely complex material that is classified by doctors as a tissue just like skin, or muscle, or bone. Now, before we go any further in our investigation into anaemia (too few red blood cells), pernicious anaemia and vitamin B_{12} deficiency, it is necessary to understand a little bit about blood.

Most people know that blood transports oxygen from the lungs to whatever cells and tissues need it – which is all of them. And even though this is an extremely important function it also does many other things:

- it removes carbon dioxide and other waste products from cells and tissue
- it supplies essential nutrients to cells including fatty acids, amino acids and glucose
- it protects us from any unwelcome organisms and infections using its arsenal of antibodies
- it regulates our acid levels

[i] An organelle is a tiny substructure with a specialised function within a cell.

- it has special cells which form clots when we bleed
- it transports hormones, which are chemicals that transmit messages telling other cells to do certain things
- it helps regulate body temperature by bringing warmth to cold parts of the body in cold weather, and by getting cooled off in the skin in hot weather
- it also has what is known as a hydraulic function – if you are a male you can thank blood for filling your penis (engorgement) when you are aroused, with the result that you experience an erection.

Blood is made up of two main component parts: cells and plasma (see Figure 1.2). Plasma is a sort of watery broth that makes up 55% of the blood volume. It consists of a solution of water (92%), proteins, lipids, inorganic ions (salts) and glucose. The proteins include hormones. The salts include urea, a waste product of cells. The cells include red blood cells (also known as erythrocytes), white blood cells (leucocytes) and platelets (thrombocytes). Take a look at Figure 1.3: the red blood cells are, well, red, the white blood cells are the round globe-like cell and the platelet is the 'cell' with the spikes. In reality, platelets are much smaller than red blood cells.[ii] Platelets form clots to stop bleeding from wounds (they are responsible for those wonderful scabs which formed on your knees when you were a child), the white blood cells combat infections and disease and the red blood cells transport oxygen around your body.

Like all human cells, red blood cells are produced in bone marrow and you produce an awful lot of them – millions and millions every day; they are the most common cells in your body. At any one time a healthy individual will have between 20 and 30 trillion red blood cells, though men will have around 5% more than women. Red blood cells 'live' in the blood for between 100 and 120 days.

[ii] Strictly speaking platelets are not cells as such, but they are counted as cells when blood is analysed.

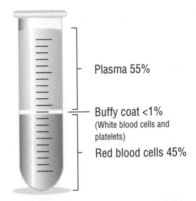

Figure 1.2 The composition of blood

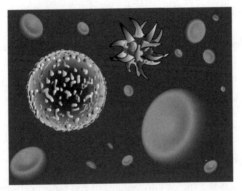

Figure 1.3 Red blood cells, white blood cells and platelets

Now that you know a little about blood – and believe me what I have just described is only a tiny amount of what has been discovered about this fascinating substance – we can turn our attention to the tricky subject of anaemia.

Anaemia

The word *anaemia* first appeared in the middle of the 19th century. It is a combination of two Greek words – *'haima'*, which means blood, and *'an'* which is Greek for 'without', so anaemia translates literally as 'without blood'. To doctors anaemia refers either to a patient not having enough red blood cells or not enough of the iron-carrying haemoglobin.

There are four causes of anaemia:

1. Inadequate production of red blood cells which could be due to:
   a. dysfunctional bone marrow – remember red blood cells are produced in bone marrow
   b. lack of B$_{12}$
   c. lack of folic acid

2. Destruction of red blood cells due to an autoimmune condition

3. Blood loss from serious injury or large surgical operations

4. Inadequate production of haemoglobin, usually because the patient is deficient in iron – see below.

Haemoglobin

Haemoglobin is the major component of red blood cells and it is what makes them red-coloured. It is made up of two essential constituent parts – a protein ('globin') and iron ('haem'). If you lack one of these two ingredients you will not be able to make haemoglobin and so you will be unable to make properly functioning red blood cells, and that would be a disaster because it is haemoglobin in red blood cells that is responsible for transporting oxygen around your body. What happens is that the iron bonds with the protein 'globin' to form haemoglobin and the oxygen then binds to the iron part of the haemoglobin. Haemoglobin then is a protein[iii] that contains four iron atoms, which is why iron is such an important part of a healthy diet; if you lack iron (iron deficiency), then it stands to reason that you won't be able to produce healthy haemoglobin. It is the haemoglobin that is responsible for transporting oxygen to wherever it is needed in the body – which is everywhere. It is easy to take oxygen for granted – it is oxygen that provides the energy to the muscles that are responsible for your eye being able to focus on this page; it is also responsible for you being able to turn the page using muscles in your fingers; it is also providing energy for your heart to keep beating; and it is even responsible for providing the energy for your brain to assimilate the printed information on this page. So, thanks to your healthy haemoglobin, you are able to carry on doing what you are doing – in short, living. Once the iron atoms have formed a bond with the oxygen, the red blood cell then goes on a remarkable journey through the arteries to wherever it is needed – your eye muscle, finger muscle ... you get the picture.

Think of the red blood cell as a bus. The bus is made of raw materials (in this case think of vitamin B_{12}), and once made it takes on board haemoglobin and sets off for the lungs. Waiting in the lungs is a queue of oxygen molecules, which hop on the bus (into the blood) where they immediately bond to the iron in the haemoglobin. The bus carries on to wherever the oxygen is needed and when it arrives, the doors open, the oxygen molecules release their grip on the haemoglobin and exit the bus. The red blood cells then return to the lungs, taking with them some waste products as they do so, although there is no 'bonding' as there was with oxygen and it's in the lungs that the whole process starts again.

So in order for the whole process of transporting oxygen through your body to function properly you will need an adequate supply of healthy red blood cells and iron. Without adequate supplies of either you will develop anaemia. Let's take a look at these two essential elements in a little more detail.

---

iii Protein in this sense is a type of large molecule and shouldn't be confused with nutritional protein.

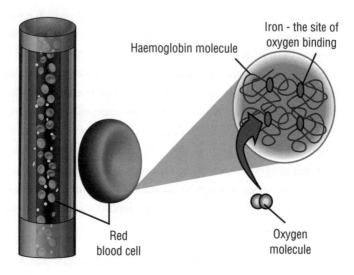

Figure 1.4 Haemoglobin

Iron

Most body stores of iron are found in a protein called *ferritin* and it is ferritin that doctors measure to deduce whether a patient has adequate levels of iron (some iron circulates in blood – serum iron). As iron is needed to combine with the globin to make healthy haemoglobin, it therefore stands to reason that a person who doesn't have enough iron stores will not be able to make haemoglobin and will therefore be anaemic – the cause of his or her anaemia will be lack of iron and the patient will be diagnosed as having 'iron-deficiency anaemia'; the lack of iron means that the haemoglobin will not be able to capture the oxygen needed. Iron deficiency is the most common nutritional deficiency in the world,[1] and in some parts of the UK it is a major problem (south Wales and north-west Scotland).[2]

Men have around 3.8 g of iron in their body and women 2.3 g. A gram is about the weight of a small paperclip so, if there is nobody watching and you have access to such paperclips, you could get an idea of how much iron you are carrying around – unless you are deficient in iron of course.

Normal ferritin levels will be determined by individual laboratories using different machines, but the average normal levels are given in Table 1.1.[3]

Table 1.1 Normal levels of ferritin

	Nanograms per millilitre (ng/ml)[a]
Men	18–270
Women	18–160
Children (6 months to 15 years)	7–140
Infants (1 to 5 months)	50–200
'Neonates' (babies, 0 to 28 days)	25–200

[a] Please note that ng/ml does not refer simply to the amount of ferritin by weight alone but to the weight in a millilitre of blood.

Take another look at the figures in Table 1.1. As you can see there is quite a wide range of 'normal' levels, especially for men (18–270 ng/ml), which means that some men will have 15 times more ferritin in their blood than others – but they would all be deemed to have 'normal' levels.

The recommended daily intake (RDI)[iv] is usually given in milligrams (mg), and according to the UK's NHS website the RDI for iron is:

- Men 8.7 mg
- Women 14.8 mg.

[iv] The recommended daily intake (RDI) has replaced the recommended daily allowance (RDA).

Women require more daily intake than men because of blood loss during menstruation.

The website also states that: 'Most people should be able to get all the iron they need by eating a varied and balanced diet,' and goes on to warn that: 'Very high doses of iron can be fatal, particularly if taken by children, so always keep iron supplements out of the reach of children,' but then states 'Taking 20 mg or less a day of iron supplements is unlikely to cause any harm.'

Iron overdose

It is possible to overdose on iron and the following are the symptoms of an iron overdose:

- constipation
- nausea
- vomiting
- stomach pain.

Why is iron deficiency so widespread and common?

It would be easy to lay the blame on our modern diet, but iron deficiency has long been a problem, with the earliest incidence of iron supplementation being recorded in 400 years BC, when the physician Melanpus added iron filings to wine to increase Persian soldiers' strength.[4] (You can still buy iron filing 'charms' that are placed in glasses of wine!) The Nihang – the ferocious Sikh warriors – will only eat food prepared in iron cooking vessels and served in iron bowls as they believe that the iron provides them with extra strength. In the UK, old pubs can be found where the wooden beams above the open fire have several scars caused by red hot pokers that had been plunged into tankards of beer – supposedly to warm the beer but it could have been to infuse the beer with iron.[v] During the Second World War the UK and US governments recommended voluntary fortification of bread with vitamins B_1, B_2, niacin and iron, the iron being obtained from worn-out railway tracks.

All of the above point to iron deficiency having been around for a long time. Any deficiency may be due to the fact that people just aren't eating enough foodstuffs that contain lots of iron and, according to the NHS's website, these foods include:

- liver
- meat
- beans
- nuts
- dried fruit, such as dried apricots
- wholegrains, such as brown rice
- fortified breakfast cereals
- soybean flour
- most dark green leafy vegetables, such as watercress and curly kale.

Anyway, let's get back on track; the fact is that to make healthy haemoglobin you need sufficient supplies of iron. And the haemoglobin will be transported around the body by healthy red blood cells. Have you noticed that whenever I have mentioned red blood cells I have always included the prefix 'healthy'? That's because, unless the red

[v] 'In a little inn, in a small village in one of the western counties of England, a group of men were assembled [in] the tap-room, where the fire was blazing very comfortably, and serving the purpose of keeping the poker at that degree of red heat necessary to warm a pot of beer when inserted therein.' (James Hannay, *King Dobbs*, 1849.)

blood cells are healthy in that they are perfectly formed, they won't be able to play their part in transporting the haemoglobin molecule[vi] It's therefore time to revisit the subject of healthy red blood cells.

Red blood cells are produced in bone marrow in all of your bones at the time of birth but by the time you reach 20 they are only produced in the flat bones – the ribs, breastbone, pelvis, cranium, shoulder blades and vertebrae – and at the ends of the long bones. And in order to produce healthy red blood cells you need adequate supplies of two important pieces of the human jigsaw: vitamin B$_{12}$ (cobalamin) and folic acid (folate). We need to know something about each of these before we continue our investigation into pernicious anaemia and vitamin B$_{12}$ deficiency. We'll begin with folate.

Folate/folic acid/B$_9$ or pteroylglutamic acid

Vitamin B$_9$ is a complex vitamin that is the subject of much heated debate on a wide range of websites and the focus of a great deal of scientific investigation. Vitamin B$_9$ can be found in its primary state as either folic acid or folate, and the first thing we need to do when discussing these two forms of vitamin B$_9$ is to clarify the differences between them.

While I have always believed that folate is the naturally occurring form of B$_9$ and that folic acid is the artificially produced form of folate, it appears that some interested parties do not agree. Here's what a recent submission to *Wikipedia* says:

> The term 'folate' is often denoted in the food supple-
> ment industry to designate 'the natural occurring form

[vi] A molecule is a group of two or more atoms, such as water, which is made up of two hydrogen atoms and one oxygen atom – hence its chemical name H$_2$O.

of folic acid'. There is no 'natural' and chemical form of folate and folic acid, and the two terms can be used interchangeably.[5]

However, this is not correct – there *is* a difference between folic acid and folate. This is how the *Designs for Health* website explains the difference:

> The terms 'folate' and 'folic acid' are often used interchangeably but they are not one and the same. Folates are members of the B vitamin family (referring to various tetrahydrofolate derivatives), naturally occurring in foods, mainly leafy green vegetables. Folic acid, on the other hand, is a fully oxidized, synthetic compound (pteroylmonoglutamic acid), used in dietary supplements and in food fortification. The important difference to note is that folic acid does not occur naturally.[6]

Some doctors believe that the synthetic form of B9 is bad for you – very bad indeed, and I will explain why in the section on fortification of flour below (see page 15). In this book I will refer to folate or folic acid as vitamin B9 even though B9 was not identified until 1941, which is why a certain Lucy Wills might have disagreed with my choice. We'll meet Miss Wills and find out more about her soon (see page 16).

What is folic acid/folate/B9?

Essentially, B9[vii] is a vitamin that has various biological functions. It naturally occurs in a wide variety of foods, including vegetables (particularly dark green leafy vegetables), fruits and fruit juices, nuts,

[vii] Also, confusingly sometimes called vitamin M, vitamin BC or folatin.

beans, peas, dairy products, poultry and meat, eggs, seafood, grains, and some beers – we'll be learning more about beer and B$_9$ soon (see page 18). Avocado, spinach, liver, yeast, asparagus and Brussels sprouts are among the foods with the highest levels of folate. That's why you should always do what your mother told you to do and 'eat your greens' (folate is named after the Latin word for leaf – *folium*).

How are levels of B$_9$ measured?

The B$_9$ status of patients is usually measured by simply examining the amount of folate in the blood – serum folate. (Actually, blood serum is part of the plasma component of blood that remains after the blood is allowed to clot and the clot is removed, along with the blood cells, by centrifugation in the lab.) The B$_9$ status of the patient can also be measured by calculating the amount of folate in red blood cells – red blood corpuscle folate.

How much B$_9$ is needed?

The United States' Food and Nutrition Board (FNB) states that:

> At least 85% of folic acid is estimated to be bioavailable when taken with food, whereas only about 50% of folate naturally present in food is bioavailable.[7]

What that means is that more folic acid will be absorbed by the patient if it is taken in tablet form than by eating food which has a high folate concentration. To address this problem the FNB developed a new way of stating the RDA – they introduced the dietary folate equivalent (DFE):

> The FNB developed DFEs to reflect the higher bioavailability of folic acid than that of food folate.[8]

14

This means that, according to the US's FNB, the DFE for both men and women should be 400 mcg (that's not a misprint). Pregnant women need 600 mcg DFE while lactating women need 500 mcg DFE. (Thankfully there are no values given for pregnant men, or men who are lactating.) According to the UK's NHS Direct website the RDA for B9 for men and women is 0.2 mg daily. Perhaps it's best just to eat your greens and get to like Marmite – more about this later (see page 17).

Folic acid fortification of flour

Quite a number of countries now add B9 to flour where it has helped to reduce, quite significantly, the number of babies born with neural tube defects, including spina bifida. At the time of writing, 76 countries in the world require at least one grain-type to be fortified with B9 and there is lively debate whether the European Union as a whole, or constituent states individually, should also follow suit. In the UK this is still being debated as there is evidence that whilst fortification has reduced the number of babies being born with a neural tube defect there are other consequences that may offset the proven benefits. One researcher outlined one of the problems like this:

> Thus, the simple interpretation is that the cognitive impairment and anemia usually associated with low vitamin B-12 status are made much worse by a high folate status.[9]

Furthermore, there is another problem with fortifying flour – it can mask one of the indicators of a B_{12} deficiency; I will explain more about this in Chapter 3.

What does B9 do?

This is a good question and one that, unfortunately for non-scientists, involves some serious biology; however, we don't need to go into this in any great depth to understand the importance of this vitamin. What we do need to know is that:

> The metabolic role of folic acid is interdependent with that of vitamin B$_{12}$ (both are required by rapidly dividing cells) and a deficiency of one may lead to deficiency of the other.[10]

The natural form of B$_9$ is tetrahydrofolate, which is usually referred to as THF; and THF is needed to produce healthy red blood cells among other things. (It plays a part in making your DNA.) So, without adequate supplies of B$_9$ you can't produce healthy red blood cells and you will suffer from folic acid anaemia. You can produce red blood cells without B$_9$, but they wouldn't be perfect and wouldn't be able to form good quality haemoglobin.

Lucy Wills, who I mentioned earlier, was a doctor and academic who was born in 1888 and was educated at Cheltenham Ladies College, the University of Cambridge (which in the second decade of the 20th century still didn't award degrees to women – she was instead issued with a Certificate) and the Royal Free Hospital in London (1920). She trained as a doctor but chose not to practise medicine, preferring to pursue a career in research and teach at the Royal Free's Department of Chemical Pathology. At this time, pregnant women were often found to be anaemic, especially those living in India. The early 1930s saw Lucy Wills investigating this phenomenon. What she found was that Indian Muslims were particularly prone to becoming anaemic when pregnant and she discovered that by feeding the women 'brewer's yeast' the anaemia was reversed. It was she who then made the link between folic acid and anaemia, even though folic acid or folate had not been identified and wouldn't be for another 10 years. Thus began the practice of ensuring that pregnant women did not become deficient in folate during their confinement by making sure they had an adequate intake of the nutrient. As a bonus, it was later found that this also reduced the risk of the baby developing neural tube defects. The brewer's yeast that Dr Wills fed to those 'poor milky creatures' was Marmite.

Brewer's yeast was invented in the late 19th century by the German scientist Justus von Liebig, who concentrated and bottled this by-product of beer making. The Marmite Food Extract Company was formed in 1902 and was based at the heart of the British brewing industry at Burton-on-Trent in Staffordshire where the Bass brewing company supplied the raw ingredients.

Marmite is full of B vitamins, which is slightly strange because there is no hint of greenness to be seen among the dark brown paste. Just one 4 g serving (about the weight of four paperclips) gives you 50% of your B9. It is also rich in vitamins B_1, B_2 and B_3 (thiamin, riboflavin and niacin respectively) and our old friend B_{12},[viii] which is why it formed part of the British soldier's rations in the First World War, a deficiency in B_1 leading to the thoroughly nasty disease of beriberi.

(Strangely, the British version of Marmite does not contain any iron whereas the Marmite produced in New Zealand does: you can get 15% of your RDA in a 5 g spread – they seem to like bigger portions in New Zealand, which might explain why their rugby team are so difficult to beat! There are other versions of Marmite produced in other countries – Vegemite and AussieMite in Australia, which are distributed to many countries, including the UK (a bit like selling sand to an Arab country), OzeMite, Cenovis (a Swiss spread) and Vegex (a yeast product available in the USA since 1913). Love it or hate it, Marmite, especially the New Zealand version, is very good for you.)

With nearly 8000 members, the Pernicious Anaemia Society has a quite a few elderly members. When they telephone the office to

---

viii Vitamin B_{12} is added to the Marmite which means that it wouldn't have been present in the early versions of the product.

enquire more about their newly diagnosed disease they almost always tell of how much of a shock it was to discover that they had pernicious anaemia because 'I eat Marmite nearly every day'. The reason that they say this is that for decades, Marmite was considered to be an essential part of the British diet. Even I can remember a poster hanging on the wall of my primary school classroom that illustrated healthy foods and gave instructions on how to achieve a healthy diet. Marmite was a prominent item, along with rose hip syrup. Today, both these products are not as popular as perhaps they should be.

Diseases and conditions leading to B$_9$ deficiency

Unfortunately, no matter how much B$_9$ you ingest, there are certain diseases and medicines that can cause a deficiency. All of the following call for extra supplies of B$_9$ and, consequently, can and do lead to a deficiency if there is no extra intake:

- malaria
- skin diseases, such as dermatitis with peeling and eczema
- Crohn's disease
- liver disorders
- coeliac disease, which is where the patient cannot digest gluten[ix] and absorb B$_9$
- kidney dialysis (it causes B$_9$ deficiency as it is excreted in urine)
- hypothyroidism (underactive thyroid)
- alcohol abuse.

As I have mentioned, some beers are a valuable contributor to a diet rich in B$_9$. However, I recommend that before you embark on a beer-based diet you discuss this with your doctor; please, be prepared to be disappointed.

[ix] From the Latin for glue – *gluten*; it's a protein found in wheat and other grains and gives elasticity to dough.

Drugs and medicines affecting B9

All of the following regularly prescribed medications adversely affect B9 storage, uptake or function:

- sulphasalazine, used to treat Crohn's disease
- trimethoprin (Septrim, Bactrim), an antibiotic used to treat bladder infections
- pyrimethamine (Daraprim), used to treat malaria
- triamterene (a diuretic, 'water tablets')
- anti-epileptics (including phenytoin, phenobarbitone and primodone), which are usually prescribed along with folic acid.

Again, the effect of these medicines on your B9 will be small despite dire statements to the contrary on various social media. You should never stop taking any medicines without first discussing this with your doctor. Ask if you should take a supplement.

Without adequate levels of B9 you will not be able to produce healthy red blood cells, but that isn't the only consequence of a deficiency in the vitamin. Symptoms include sore tongue, weakness, headaches, heart palpitations, irritability and behavioural disorders. We shall see later on that there have been some studies where B9 has been successful in treating a wide range of psychiatric illnesses, including depression.

Before we finish with the B9 it is worth noting that B9 should never be used to treat any vitamin B_{12} deficiency without first addressing B_{12} levels. If a person is low in B_{12}, for whatever reason, his or her deficiency should be addressed and corrected first. Trying to correct any B_{12} deficiency with B9 will only lead to the patient becoming even more deficient in B_{12}.

Having mentioned that caveat, it's now time to examine the other key player in the production of healthy red blood cells, the most complex of all vitamins and the only vitamin that has a metal at its core – vitamin B$_{12}$, otherwise known as cobalamin. An introduction like that should be accompanied by a round of applause, don't you think?

Vitamin B$_{12}$

I have a particular affection for vitamin B$_{12}$. The reason for this bonding between us is probably due to the fact that for a good few years I had next to none of it in my body and, if the old adage is to be believed, absence makes the heart grow fonder. I certainly missed it, so when we were at last reunited we formed a different, more intense relationship; more of this later.

Vitamin B$_{12}$ is the second main protagonist in the production of healthy red blood cells. Without adequate supplies of this vitamin any red cells that are produced will be of poor quality in that they will often be enlarged or 'stretched' and won't be able to accommodate the iron and, as a consequence, the oxygen. Vitamin B$_{12}$ was discovered, or rather isolated, in 1947 and was first known as 'anti-intrinsic factor' for reasons that we will discover later.

What is vitamin B$_{12}$?

Vitamin B$_{12}$ is one of the eight B vitamins and there are, for our purposes, four different types of B$_{12}$. Each type is actually a *cobalamin* because at the core of the chemical structure lies the somewhat rare metal cobalt.

Vitamin B$_{12}$ can only be made by bacteria. Many animals, cows and horses included, have bacteria that produce B$_{12}$ in their stomachs. Humans obtain it from animal products, such as dairy, meat, fish and shellfish, that have already made or produced the vitamin.

Sources of B$_{12}$

Other than 'artificial' B$_{12}$, we humans obtain our B$_{12}$ from any animal product as stated above. Not all animal products have the same amounts of B$_{12}$, with liver and other offal providing the highest concentrations. Yet just because certain products contain lots of B$_{12}$, some foodstuffs are better at yielding them or giving them up so to speak. Dairy products are far more willing to let you extract their B$_{12}$ than meat is, for example.[11]

The four distinct types of B$_{12}$ are:

- **Hydroxocobalamin** ($C_{62}H_{89}CoN_{13}O_{15}P$: OHCbl) – This is considered to be more 'active' and 'purer' than cyanocobalamin (see next) and is actually produced by fermenting bacteria.

- **Cyanocobalamin** ($C_{63}H_{88}CoN_{14}O_{14}Pn$: CNCbl) – This is produced by passing hydroxocobalamin over *activated charcoal*[x] and adding cyanide to it and so, yes, it does contain a very small, but some would say significant, amount of cyanide. It is the most common form of artificial B$_{12}$ (or some would say semi-artificial because it is 'grown') and France is the biggest producer (80% of the world's production). Over half (55%) of all cyanocobalamin 'grown' or produced ends up in animal feeds, with 45% destined for humans,[12] most of which is added to fortified foods, such as breakfast cereals and multivitamin pills. (Take a look at the ingredients of your daily multivitamin and it will almost always state that the B$_{12}$ is in the form of cyanocobalamin.) So, because cyanocobalamin is actually hydroxocobalamin that has been purified to a certain extent, it can be regarded as a purer, though more processed, form of B$_{12}$.

---

[x] Carbon that has been processed so that it has very small 'pores' that absorb certain toxins.

- **Methylcobalamin** (C$_{63}$H$_{91}$CoN$_{13}$O$_{14}$P: MeCbl) – This is based on cyanocobalamin but methyl iodine replaces the cyanide. This is considered to be an 'active' form of B$_{12}$. There is some evidence that it is effective in treating peripheral neuropathy and diabetic neuropathy.[13] Unlike hydroxocobalamin and cyanocobalamin, it is not licensed in the UK or North America, which doesn't stop 10% of members of the Pernicious Anaemia Society using it to treat their condition.[14] (It's the type I use – 5 mg/ml to be exact twice a week using small disposable single-use syringes.)

- **Adenosylcobalamin** (C$_{72}$H$_{100}$CoN$_{18}$O$_{17}$P: AdoCbl) – This was, until relatively recently, believed to be unstable, meaning that it didn't last very long. However, in recent years it has been produced in a stable form and a recent quick internet search showed that it is readily available as sub-lingual drops, sub-lingual tablets, oral tablets and injections. This is the 'purest' form of naturally occurring B$_{12}$ and is currently the subject of much debate among interested scientists.

Methylation

We could get bogged down in some very complex biochemistry here, but I'll keep it simple as much for my sake as for yours. Basically, both cyanocobalamin and hydroxocobalamin have to be converted into methylcobalamin as methylcobalamin is the only form of B$_{12}$ that can take part in the complex biochemistry that results in the production of healthy red blood cells. This process is called the 'methylation cycle' and the end result is that the bone marrow is able to do its job of producing healthy red blood cells and the amount of a substance called homocysteine produced by the body is regulated. That's why I use methylcobalamin: why would I want to go through the trouble of converting the hydroxocobalamin or cyanocobalamin into methylcobalamin when somebody wearing a white coat in a laboratory has already done it for me? We'll come back to the methylation cycle in more detail later on (see pages 164-5).

How is B_{12} measured?

Whilst there are other 'markers' of B_{12} deficiency, the way in which a patient's B_{12} status is assessed by doctors is by looking at just how much B_{12} is in the patient's serum (again, the blood plasma with the clotting agents removed). Deficiency thresholds are troublesome – really troublesome – and are the cause of a great deal of frustration and ill-health. We will look at this issue soon (see page 92).

How much B_{12} is needed?

A normal healthy person needs 2.4 mcg of B_{12} every day. If he or she exceeds that the consequence is – nothing. You cannot overdose on B_{12} as it is water soluble and you just wee any excess away – something that should be more widely appreciated.

Science recap

Before we go on to examine just what pernicious anaemia is, now's a good time to sum up what we have learned.

- Anaemia can mean the patient has insufficient red blood cells or low haemoglobin.
- Haemoglobin, present in red blood cells, is a molecule made up of a protein (globin), iron and oxygen.
- Red blood cells are produced in bone marrow and require healthy levels of iron, B_{12} and folate (B_9) to form properly.
- B_{12} is found in animal products and folate is found in some animal products and leafy vegetables.

So, if a normal person has adequate supplies of folate and iron, then he or she will be producing healthy red blood cells that, courtesy of the haemoglobin they contain, will be able to transport oxygen to wherever it is needed and get rid of waste products without even having to think about it. He or she will *not* be suffering from anaemia – ah, happy days.

Pernicious anaemia

I used to have pernicious anaemia. There was a time, back in the day, when I was severely anaemic and left undiagnosed and untreated for several years. The anaemia would eventually have caused my death – that's what the 'pernicious' part means, *ruinous, destructive and fatal.* Following two, maybe three, years of ill-health I was finally diagnosed and treated and the anaemia was corrected – the full, heartbreaking story can be found in my first book (you really should get it); mine is regrettably not an isolated case. Unfortunately, I have been left with permanent nerve damage due to the length of time taken to diagnose and treat me. I also still have some, if not all, of the original symptoms, but that's another story – an abbreviated version of my story appears in Appendix 1.

Do I still have pernicious anaemia? It's an interesting question given my continuing symptoms, because as I am typing this my red blood cells are healthy and carrying haemoglobin and oxygen around my body. I am therefore not anaemic. However, the reason why my red blood cells are healthy is because I receive injections of vitamin B$_{12}$. Consequently, should I stop receiving injections then I would once again be unable to make healthy red blood cells and would gradually become anaemic and eventually die. So, right now I don't have anaemia that will prove pernicious, but this is only because I receive replacement vitamin B$_{12}$ replacement therapy injections. I'll explain why this is so.

I became anaemic because I couldn't produce healthy red blood cells; mine were, at the time of my diagnosis, ridiculously large and incapable of carrying much oxygen. And the reason why I was unable to produce healthy red blood cells was because I was unable to extract vitamin B_{12} from the food I ate, even though this included lots of animal products. Now, the reason why I couldn't absorb B_{12} from food was because there was, and is, something wrong with part of my digestive system. That is what sets pernicious anaemia apart from other forms of anaemia. If you are anaemic because you don't have enough B_9 in your diet, you can just up your intake of all things folate (or pop some folic acid in your mouth). Similarly, if you have inadequate supplies of iron, you can increase the amount of iron in your diet, or take an iron pill, and your deficiency will be corrected and production of healthy red blood cells containing sufficient haemoglobin will resume.

The problem with the absorption, or rather lack of absorption, of B_{12} is not due to a problem with my blood; it's all to do with issues with my digestive process which I will now attempt to describe in a clear and concise way. There is a more detailed description of the full digestive process in – well, I'll leave you to guess where you will find it.

A normal healthy person will have, in the lining of their stomach, strange little cells called gastric parietal cells. These parietal cells produce an important protein called *intrinsic factor*. Intrinsic factor was first identified, or explained, in the late 1920s by a Doctor Castle, who used to treat his pernicious anaemia patients by regurgitating raw hamburgers and feeding these to them; his patients did not know what it was they were eating, but they made a remarkable recovery. This demonstrated that there was *something* in the stomach that made all the difference. The intrinsic factor produced in the stomach makes its way, with food that is being digested, through the small intestine. This is made up of three parts – the duodenum, the jejunum and the ileum (see Figure 1.5). Most nutrients from food are absorbed in the jejunum, but iron is absorbed in the duodenum and our friend B$_{12}$ is absorbed in the last part of the small intestine – the ileum. In the ileum a bit of chemical magic takes place. The intrinsic factor binds to the B$_{12}$, that by this time has been freed from the food which carried it to the ileum (the food is the *extrinsic factor* by the way), to make a mixture of B$_{12}$ and intrinsic factor known as 'B$_{12}$ /IF complex'. This allows B$_{12}$ to then enter cells on the wall of the ileum after binding to receptors on the surface of the

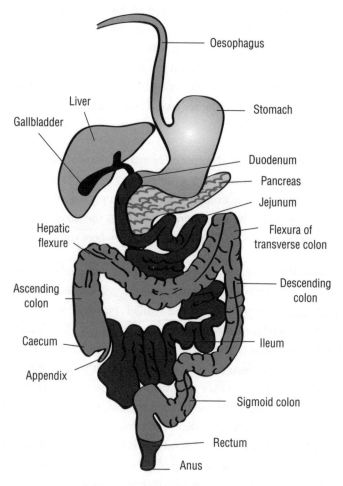

Figure 1.5 The digestive system

ileal cells; from there it passes into the blood stream. It then goes on to play its part in producing healthy red blood cells.

Now for the sad bit; people who have traditional pernicious anaemia either do not produce any intrinsic factor in their stomach or, as is the case with me, do produce intrinsic factor but at the same time, for reasons unknown, produce an antibody that destroys it. When this happens the patient is diagnosed as having 'autoimmune pernicious anaemia'. I therefore have an autoimmune disease; I also have one other – psoriasis.

Other autoimmune diseases include alopecia, coeliac disease, type 1 diabetes and Hashimoto's thyroiditis. Doctors don't know why in these diseases the patient's body seems to attack itself, but if a patient has one autoimmune condition the chances are that he or she will also have others. Thankfully, I have just two.

Pernicious anaemia and B_{12} deficiency

I am often told that as the Chairman of the Pernicious Anaemia Society I should also be campaigning for all of those who have B_{12} deficiency and not just for those whose deficiency is caused by pernicious anaemia. However, this is a complicated issue revolving around the definition of pernicious anaemia. For example, let's take the case of a patient who has had part of their ileum removed (an ileostomy – see page 51). As we have seen above, the magical process whereby the B_{12}/IF complex enters the patient's bloodstream takes place in the ileum. So if a patient has undergone an ileostomy then he or she won't be able to absorb B_{12} and will need replacement B_{12} therapy for life. If that patient didn't receive injections of B_{12} he or she would go on to develop anaemia because of the inability to produce healthy red blood cells, which would eventually prove fatal – so does he or she have pernicious anaemia or just the potential to develop pernicious anaemia? It's an interesting question but one that I haven't been able to find a definitive answer to. Suffice it to say that if a patient has B_{12}-deficiency anaemia for reasons other than poor diet, the issues discussed in this book will all be relevant.

Summary

In this chapter we have examined, in quite some detail, how oxygen is transported throughout the body. We've looked at the role of B_{12}, folate and iron in making healthy red blood cells that are capable of allowing oxygen transportation, and we have seen why patients that have pernicious anaemia are unable to absorb vitamin B_{12} from food. It is now time to move on, in the next chapter, to discuss the causes and consequences of vitamin B_{12} deficiency in general.

References

1   Centers for Disease Control and Prevention. Iron deficiency – United States, 1999–2000. *Morbidity and Mortality Weekly Report* 2002; 51:899.

2   Gomez J. *How to Cope with Anaemia*. London, Sheldon Press: 1998.

3   WebMD. *Ferritin*. www.webmd.com/a-to-z-guides/ferritin?page=2 (Accessed 27 November 2014).

4   Kamien M. The repeating history of objections to the fortifica-tion of bread and alcohol: from iron filings to folic acid. *Medical Journal of Australia* 2006; 184(12):638-640.

5   Wikipedia. Folic acid. http://en.wikipedia.org/wiki/Folic_acid (Accessed 29 November 2014).

6   Designs for Health. Folic acid vs folate Part 1. http://blog.de-signsforhealth.com/blog/bid/115121/Folic-Acid-vs-Folate-Part-I (Accessed 29 November 2014).

7   National Institutes of Health. Folate Dietary Supplement Fact Sheet. http://ods.od.nih.gov/factsheets/Folate-HealthProfessional/

(accessed 30 November 2014).

8   Ibid.

9   Smith AD. Folic acid fortification: the good, the bad, and the puzzle of vitamin B-12. *American Journal of Clinical Nutrition* 2007; 85(1):3–5.

10 *Oxford Concise Colour Medical Dictionary* Fourth edition. Oxford, Oxford University Press: 2007.

11 Vogiatzoglou A, Smith AD, Nurk E, Berstad P, Drevon CA, Ueland PM, Vollset SE, Tell GS, Refsum H. Dietary sources of vitamin B-12 and their association with plasma vitamin B-12 concentrations in the general population: the Hordaland Homocysteine Study 1-3. *American Journal of Clinical Nutrition* 2009; 89:1078–1087.

12 Kaesler B. Vitamins: B9. Vitamin B_{12} (Cyanocobalamins). *Ullmann's Encyclopedia of Industrial Chemistry*. Weinheim, Wiley-VCH: 2005.

13 Izumi Y, Kaji R. Clinical trials of ultra-high-dose methylcobalamin in ALS. *Brain Nerve* 2007; 59(10):1141–1147.

14 Hooper M, Hudson P, Porter F, McCaddon A. Patients' journeys: the diagnosis and treatment of pernicious anaemia. *British Journal of Nursing* 2014; 23(7):16-24.

Chapter 2

Causes of vitamin B$_{12}$ deficiency

In the previous chapter we saw how important vitamin B$_{12}$ is to good health, so it might come as some surprise for you to know that vitamin B$_{12}$ deficiency is a serious worldwide problem. Given that any B$_{12}$ deficiency will lead to the patient experiencing a wide range of symptoms that can make everyday living difficult, at best, and, at worst, debilitating, this worldwide problem is causing unnecessary suffering that warrants global investigation. In this chapter I will first try to establish how widespread and prevalent B$_{12}$ deficiency is and then look at the various causes of this problem.

Prevalence of B$_{12}$ deficiency?

The *British Journal of Medicine* in the autumn of 2014 stated:

> In the United Kingdom and United States the prevalence
> of vitamin B$_{12}$ deficiency is around 6% in people aged less
> than 60 years, and closer to 20% in those aged more than 60
> years.[1]

It's all too easy to take those figures in a carefree and even nonchalant manner, but let's put some meat on the bones of these percentages.

In the UK, according to the 2011 census, there are 14,183,000 people over the age of 60:[2] 20% of that figure means that 2,836,600 people living in the UK over the age of 60 will be deficient in this essential vitamin – that's nearly three million. Again, if you look at the figures involved in those *under* the age of 60 (6% of 48,999,000) the figure is again nearly three million (2,939,000). So, in the UK population as a whole, nearly six million people will be deficient in vitamin B$_{12}$; in other words, nearly six million people are going about their daily lives suffering, to some extent or another, from the consequences of having less than an optimum amount of B$_{12}$ in their system.

In the United States, 18.5% of the population is over the age of 60, which, based on a total population of 308,745,538,[3] means that there are 57,117,924 people over the age of 60; and if the figures given above are to be believed, then 20% of them have a vitamin B$_{12}$ deficiency – that's a staggering 11,423,584 Americans over the age of 60 are living with an essential vitamin deficiency; and 15,097,656 of those living in the US under the age of 60 will also have a deficiency. That means that over 26.5 million Americans are suffering from B$_{12}$ deficiency.

And it gets worse – like most developed countries, both the UK and the USA are becoming very good at keeping elderly people alive and so have an ageing population; this means that in the UK the figure of nearly three million people over the age of 60 being deficient in B$_{12}$ will increase considerably in the next few years.

These are truly astounding figures, made even more astonishing considering how widely available and inexpensive supplements in the form of tablets are, that most breakfast cereals are fortified with the vitamin and that B$_{12}$ is almost always included in any of the multivitamin tablets that are consumed in their millions every day. Imagine what percentage of the population would be deficient in B$_{12}$ if fortification was not so widespread; those figures of 6% and 20% would most likely increase significantly.

Being deficient in B_{12} often, though not always, means that the sufferer will experience a wide range of symptoms (see Appendix 2), some of which are sometimes not considered by the medical profession to be associated with B_{12}. It makes me wonder how many of these patients have been told that the symptoms that they are experiencing are due to some other medical condition? How many are consequently receiving expensive and unnecessary medication? The answer is likely to run to many millions, maybe billions worldwide.

And if you think things are bad in the UK and USA, it's far worse in many other parts of the world:

> Across Latin America, approximately 40% of children and adults have clinical or sub-clinical deficiency. The prevalence of deficiency is much higher in African and Asian countries—for example, 70% in Kenyan schoolchildren, 80% in Indian pre-school children, and 70% in Indian adults.[4]

I've quickly worked out that there are 837,320,000 adults in India (over the age of 15) which means that 586,124,000 Indian adults are deficient in B_{12} – that's over half a billion people.[5] The rest of this chapter looks at the underlying cause or causes for this worldwide problem.

Pernicious anaemia

As we have already discussed in the previous chapter, patients who become deficient in B_{12} will be unable to produce healthy red blood cells – they will produce some but they will be enlarged and a strange shape and they won't last very long. When red blood cells become enlarged they are said to be 'megaloblastic'. Contrary to what many doctors believe, not all patients with serious B_{12} deficiency will have megaloblastic red blood cells – but more of this later. However, let's begin with looking at the role of pernicious anaemia: 'PA is the major cause of severe megaloblastic anemia in the world.'[6]

As we have seen, patients with pernicious anaemia are unable to absorb the essential vitamin B$_{12}$ from food because their bodies destroy the protein that makes the absorption possible – the intrinsic factor. So how common is pernicious anaemia? It's impossible to say because of the problems with diagnosing it but some clinicians (Andres and Serraj) have made a brave attempt: 'Its prevalence is 0.1% in the general population and 1.9% in subjects over the age of 60 years.'[7]

That figure is almost certainly wildly inaccurate for three reasons.

- **Firstly**, there are no accurate and reliable figures on how many people are diagnosed with pernicious anaemia – or at least I have not been able to identify any such data set. So no record is kept of how many people receive a firm diagnosis.

- **Secondly**, misdiagnosis is so prevalent that if such a data set does exist it will not include the enormous number of patients who are wrongly diagnosed in the first place. The results of the Pernicious Anaemia Society's survey showed that 44% of patients were wrongly diagnosed before finally being told the correct cause of their symptoms: 'Before the final diagnosis of pernicious anaemia was made, respondents were asked if they were incorrectly given another explanation for their symptoms. 50% said "No", 44% said "Yes" and the remaining 6% did not answer.'[8] So, 44% of patients were originally told that their symptoms were attributable to some other illness, and what a wide range of often exotic illnesses they were and we'll discuss this in Chapter 4. The point I'm making is that even if there is a record of just how many people receive a diagnosis of having pernicious anaemia, the figures will only account for just over half of people who have the condition with the other half being told that they have something other than pernicious anaemia, often for many years.

- **Thirdly**, a great many patients will be told that they have a B_{12} deficiency and, because the test for the anti-intrinsic factor antibody is flawed, and because the treatment will be the same whether the deficiency is caused by full-blown pernicious anaemia or not, no further tests are carried out leaving the patient in a kind of no-mans-land – receiving treatment but not having a firm diagnosis. I don't have any figures to support this, but I know from the telephone calls and visits to the Pernicious Anaemia Society's offices that it is more widespread than is generally acknowledged.

All of this means that the statement by Andres and Serraj that 'pernicious anaemia is prevalent in 0.1% in the general population and 1.9% in subjects over the age of 60 years' is a brave attempt to put some figures together – but they should be taken with a great big pinch of salt. On the other hand the figures at least give us something to go on. More reliable is what Professor Andres and Dr Serraj go on to say about the total percentage of patients whose B_{12} deficiency is due to them having pernicious anaemia: 'Pernicious anemia represents 20%–50% of the causes of vitamin B_{12} deficiency in adults.'

So, there we have it – pernicious anaemia is the cause of B_{12} deficiency in 20–50% of patients – which is pretty meaningless really as the range is so great. Other researchers disagree, and it is probably safer to say that pernicious anaemia is the biggest cause of vitamin B_{12} deficiency in developed countries, malnutrition is more likely to be the main cause in less-developed countries; but what we can be certain of is that pernicious anaemia is one of the leading, if not the main, causes of vitamin B_{12} deficiency – at least in the developed world. The difficulty here is that because there are so many problems in diagnosing pernicious anaemia, any statistics are going to be an underestimation. Still, let's just agree that pernicious anaemia, whether diagnosed or not, is the biggest cause of B_{12} deficiency in the developed world. And now it's time to look at the other causes of any deficiency.

Diet

One spring morning in the 1770s Dr Richard Price, mathematician, philosopher and theologian was taking a walk in the fields near his house and chapel in Bethnal Green, London. As was usual for this celebrated figure of the time he was deep in thought as he made his way through the countryside. Suddenly he came across many larks that had been trapped in a net by some hunters. Upset by the obvious distress the larks were in he quickly set about freeing them. He carried on with his walk and then realised that those larks were nourishment for some poor family and so he returned to the site of the net and deposited some money in order that the family might eat that day.

Larks, you see, were an important source of free meat. Even though there isn't much flesh on the birds it would have provided *some* nourishment, especially in the form of B_{12}. I mention this because eating foodstuffs that contain B_{12} was seen as essential long before any vitamins had been discovered. In the ancient world larks provided a free source of protein and of B_{12}, alongside rabbits, doves, rats and a now much neglected source of B_{12} – wall fish, otherwise known as snails (0.5 mg per snail). Before animal husbandry became established, people would eat all manner of B_{12}-rich foods, including cheese, butter and eggs, without knowing why these were an essential part of their diet and a basic building-block for good health. And this is my way of introducing one of the much talked about ways in which people can become deficient in B_{12} – through their diet.

I believe it is extremely difficult to become deficient in B_{12} through diet alone, though I realise it is not impossible. It is usually stated that B_{12} is only available from food that is of animal origin and, yes, this used to be the case. However, since the introduction of artificially produced B_{12} the vitamin is to be found in every pharmacy, supermarket and health store. And fortification of foodstuffs is now so widespread that you would have to try hard to become deficient; it comes as some surprise to discover that B_{12} deficiency is so prevalent.

> In the UK in 1980, the average time taken to prepare the evening meal was 90 minutes, which fell to 30 minutes in the 1990s and was recently measured at 20 minutes. Whilst the time spent on preparing meals has decreased there has been a corresponding rise in the number of cookery books available and the number of cookery programmes on television.

One group of people who are obviously at risk of developing a deficiency are strict vegetarians and vegans. According to the Department for the Environment, Food and Rural Affairs, vegans make up 2% of the population and within this group the prevalence of vitamin B_{12} deficiency ranges from 47.8% to as high as 86.5% in strict vegans.[9] In other words, between half and over three quarters of vegans will be deficient in B_{12}, which is an astonishingly high figure considering that vegans will surely be aware of the danger of becoming deficient in B_{12} if they follow their chosen lifestyle without using supplements. For whatever reason, over half of vegans are not ensuring that they have an adequate supply of B_{12}.

What about the rest of the population who are not vegetarians or vegans? Could they be deficient in B_{12}? Well, it's unlikely to be due to their diet because, although we are eating less meat, especially red meat, than before, and because offal, which is especially rich in B_{12}, is not as popular as it once was (when did you last have braised lamb's heart?), a wide range of modern foodstuffs is fortified with not only iron and calcium but also with B_{12} and folic acid.

Fortification

There is a healthy debate taking place over whether or not the UK should follow the US and Canada and fortify all flours with folic acid. However, fortification of flour with calcium and iron is not a new idea. It was originally called for in the UK during the Second World War because some foods that were high in calcium and iron were unavailable due to rationing.

> Today foods are commonly fortified to restore levels of nu-
> trients lost during storage, handling and manufacture, and
> for the purpose of enrichment, irrespective of their original
> nutrient levels, as would be the case for the fortification of
> foods (namely flour) with folic acid – a debate that has been
> on the public health agenda for over 15 years. Mandatory
> Fortification of flour for white and brown flours with iron
> (along with thiamine and nicotinic acid)^i was introduced
> in 1956 as a means of ensuring the nutrient quality of the
> grains in refined flours. However, despite a decrease in the
> amount of bread consumed, cereals continue to provide
> over 50% of the iron in the diet because of the voluntary
> fortification of breakfast cereals. Breakfast cereals account
> for approximately 20% of the total intake of iron.[10]

So whereas we used to eat foods rich in B$_{12}$ for breakfast – bacon, eggs and sausages as a matter of course – during the 20th century the more convenient breakfast cereals, which required far less prepara-tion, became increasingly popular. And they are an ideal food to be fortified with all manner of vitamins and minerals. Take a look at the nutritional information panel on the box or packet that contain the corn flakes you have for breakfast – you'll be surprised what has been added to those little golden flakes. Interestingly the first

---

^{i} Vitamin B$_1$ and vitamin B$_3$ respectively. Nicotinic acid is a form of niacin – B$_3$.

breakfast cereals were introduced to prevent constipation and one of the original cereals was sold with the promise that 'it'll make your red blood redder.'

Naturally occurring B_{12}

The foods that contain the most B_{12} are:

- cooked clams (100 g gets you 1,648% of your daily value)
- beef liver (100 g provides 1,386% of your daily value)
- All-Bran (100 g provides 333% of your daily value)
- red meat (beef) (100 g provides 100% of your daily value)

and remember, 100 g is not a lot – think of 100 little paper clips.

There is one last area to discuss in relation to B_{12} sources – the problem with food production rich in B_{12}. Beef in particular and meat in general is expensive to produce not only in economic terms but also in environmental terms – it takes 15,000 kg of water to produce 1 kg of beef[11] which for many scientists is simply not sustainable. So what of future sources of B_{12}? Well, though there might be a problem in producing enough 'natural' B_{12} we can always turn to supplements that can be taken in various forms, or we can turn to the dietary saviours of the future – insects.

Future sources of B_{12}

In 2013 the Food and Agriculture Organisation of the United Nations published its report on the use of insects as a source of food in the report 'Edible insects: future prospects for food and feed security'.[12] The report addressed a really serious problem that the world faces – we are running out of food and the report begins with a dire warning:

It is widely accepted that by 2050 the world will host 9 billion people. To accommodate this number, current food production will need to almost double. Land is scarce and expanding the area devoted to farming is rarely a viable or sustainable option. Oceans are overfished and climate change and related water shortages could have profound implications for food production. To meet the food and nutrition challenges of today – there are nearly 1 billion chronically hungry people worldwide – and tomorrow, what we eat and how we produce it needs to be re-evaluated. Inefficiencies need to be rectified and food waste reduced. We need to find new ways of growing food.

The report identifies insects as being the saviour and advocates the development of insect farms on a gigantic scale so that we can all benefit from the nutritional benefits of these charming creatures. And a certain Mark D Finke has taken the time to analyse the nutritional value of a wide range of insects[13] including determining the vitamin B$_{12}$ content of individual creepy-crawlies. Whilst moths and butterflies contain very little B$_{12}$ (*Imbrasia epimethea* – members of a family of moths from Africa contains only 0.2 mcg per kg) others are quite rich in B$_{12}$ – *Acheta domesticus* (known more commonly as the house cricket) can provide you with 174.3 mcg per kg, which means to ingest the RDI of 2.4 mcg you would need only eat 140 g of the crickets to get your daily intake. The tables are quite remarkable, with some entries stating that the insect had had its hair removed before being analysed – and you thought peeling Brussels sprouts was a chore.

The strange case of seaweed

Meanwhile, it seems there is a possible vegetarian source of B$_{12}$. Until recently it was assumed that, although seaweed is a good source of iodine and iron, the B$_{12}$ it contained was of an inactive form – it contained analogues of B_{12}. Now scientists know that two particular types of seaweed – dried green laver (*Enteromorpha sp.*) and purple laver (*Porphyra sp.*) – contain significant amounts of B_{12}, which makes them a suitable food for vegetarians.[14] Nori, which is dried purple laver, is used extensively in Japanese sushi dishes and the Welsh delicacy laverbread is also made from purple laver. I recently sent off a few tins of the seaweed to a team of researchers in Japan who have carried out a series of experiments to determine whether it contains any B_{12} and surprise, surprise, it does contain decent amounts of 'active' B_{12}. Another surprising source of B_{12} for vegetarians is shiitake mushrooms, although the actual amount in the fungi varies considerably.

The importance of 'bioavailability'

Mention of 'inactive' and 'active' forms of B_{12} brings us to another important point. Just because certain foods have high concentrations of B_{12} it doesn't mean that they are the best sources of the vitamin. This is because fish and dairy products 'give up' the vitamin more readily than meat and eggs,[15] meaning that the B_{12} found in fish and dairy products is said to be more 'bio-available'.

A person who eats a balanced diet (and that doesn't mean eating five portions of fruit or vegetable every day – there's no B_{12} in fruit or vegetables) will ingest enough B_{12} to prevent any deficiency, even if we once consumed more B_{12} rich foods than we do now. So, although some people will have a deficiency caused by diet (think of all those on the Indian sub-continent who do not eat animal products) there has to be another explanation why B_{12} deficiency is so widespread other than being caused by pernicious anaemia or diet, and it is to these causes that we will now turn.

Gastric atrophy

Atrophy is the medical term for the 'wasting away' of parts of the body. Atrophy can be caused by *apoptosis*, which is where cells simply die due to any one of a number of reasons, including advancing age. Gastric atrophy is the result of chronic inflammation of the lining of the stomach, which leads to the stomach lining not being able to do what it is supposed to do – produce hydrochloric acid (that helps to break down food), pepsin (which is an enzyme[ii] that helps break down protein in food into peptides), and our old friend intrinsic factor. Symptoms of chronic gastritis include bloating, belching, stomach pains, nausea and sometimes vomiting and black stools. People who have gastric atrophy stand a 10–20% risk of developing peptic ulcers during their lifetime and a 1–2% of developing stomach cancer.[16] There are two main causes of gastric atrophy (sometimes called atrophic gastritis): *Helicobacter pylori* and autoimmune gastritis.

Helicobacter pylori

Helicobacter pylori is a bacterium that lives in the stomach and at least half the world's population is infected by it, making it the most widespread infection in the world.[17] It is more common in the developing world than in developed industrial countries – it's estimated that 25% of the population of the developed world are infected. Surprisingly around 85% of patients who are infected never experience any of the symptoms listed above. The bacteria burrow into the lining of the stomach, thus escaping the hydrochloric acid that usually destroys any unwelcome visitors.

[ii] An enzyme is a protein molecule that helps speed up biological processes by acting as a catalyst. Enzymes are responsible for some laundry products being 'biological' in that they help speed up the process of stain removal.

Autoimmune gastritis

This is the true cause of pernicious anaemia – *autoimmune metaplastic atrophic gastritis* to give it its full name (abbreviated to AMAG). AMAG occurs when the patient produces antibodies that destroy either the parietal cells in the stomach which are the cells that produce intrinsic factor, or allow the parietal cells to do their job but produce an antibody that destroys any intrinsic factor made by the cells. Some patients make extra sure that their stomach doesn't play an active part in their health by producing parietal cell antibodies and intrinsic factor antibodies – a real double whammy. By doing this the patient doesn't allow the stomach to do what it is supposed to do and the result is a lack of intrinsic factor which, as we saw in the last chapter, is responsible for absorbing vitamin B_{12} from food (animal products). This lack of intrinsic factor means the patient will have pernicious anaemia. Nobody knows why some people unwittingly destroy parts of their own biological processes but we do know that there is a genetic link which is why many members of the Pernicious Anaemia Society have family members who have also been diagnosed with the disease. The results of the Pernicious Anaemia Society's survey confirm this: 15% of respondents reported a parent had been diagnosed with pernicious anaemia, 15% a grandparent, 9% an uncle or aunt with the condition and 2% had a child who also had been diagnosed as having pernicious anaemia.

In addition to being unable to absorb dietary vitamin B_{12} from food, patients with pernicious anaemia are also unable to reabsorb vitamin B_{12} secreted in bile. This is what is known as the *enterohepatic circulation* of B_{12}. Any unused B_{12} usually gets absorbed back into the liver where it passes into another part of the small intestine via the bile duct. Biliary secretion of vitamin B_{12} is estimated to be between 0.3 and 0.5 mcg/day.[18] So even if a person didn't eat any animal product for a significant amount of time, the re-circulating B_{12} would mean that he or she wouldn't experience the symptoms of

B$_{12}$ deficiency for some considerable time because he or she would be recycling the B$_{12}$ that they did have.

> Interruption of this so-called enterohepatic circulation of vitamin B$_{12}$ causes the body to go into a significant negative balance for the vitamin. Although the body typically has sufficient vitamin B$_{12}$ stores to last 3–5 years, once PA has been established the lack of absorption of new vitamin B$_{12}$ is compounded by the loss of the vitamin because of negative balance. When the stores have been depleted, the final stages of deficiency are often quite rapid, resulting in death in a period of months if left untreated.[19]

To sum up then, one of the causes of vitamin B$_{12}$ deficiency is gastric atrophy which is caused either by *Helicobacter pylori* or by autoimmune metaplastic atrophic gastritis which is more commonly known as full-blown autoimmune pernicious anaemia. However, there are yet more causes of B$_{12}$ deficiency, one of which is not very pleasant at all – worms.

Parasites

Fish tapeworm

Many cultures eat raw fish, including sushi and sashimi in Japanese cuisine, tartare maison in French-speaking populations, ceviche in Latin American cuisine, carpaccio di persico in Italian and marinated herring in Scandinavia. And by eating raw fish there is always the danger of you acquiring a worm who will come to live in your small intestine for up to 20 years, where it could grow to over 30 feet in length – introducing Mr Diphyllobothrium.[iii] Mr D, otherwise known as the broad fish tapeworm, has its eggs ingested by small crustaceans, which are then eaten by small fish such as minnows, which are then eaten by larger fish such as trout, perch or pike, which can then pass on the worm to humans if it is not destroyed by cooking. The eggs can also be deposited in the faeces of animals that have eaten raw fish – bears, for example. Mr D loves vitamin B_{12}, stealing up to 80% of its host's intake and thereby causing a B_{12} deficiency.

Would the patient have true pernicious anaemia if he/she were not infested by this worm? Well, the patient would have normally functioning parietal cells and would produce intrinsic factor without producing any antibodies to destroy the intrinsic factor. When Dr Castle started to keep patients alive by eating raw hamburgers, regurgitating them once they had mixed with the gastric juices in his stomach (which will have contained intrinsic factor) and then fed them to patients either orally or by a tube going into their stomach, he demonstrated that the patients were lacking any intrinsic factor. But if you tried feeding regurgitated raw hamburger meat to patients with a fish tapeworm, the worm would absorb the mixture without saying thank you.

> *Diphyllobothrium latum*, attached to the proximal portion
> (jejunum) of the intestine, absorbs the vitamin B_{12} contained
> in the food, thus preventing vitamin bound to the intrinsic
> factor of the gastric juice from reaching the receptors in the
> distal portions of the small intestine of the host. In genuine
> pernicious anaemia, remission results from the administra-
> tion of vitamin B_{12} + gastric juice both by mouth and into the
> ileum.[20]

So the patient with *Diphyllobothrium* infestation would have a B_{12} deficiency but that deficiency would be caused by the tapeworm and not by pernicious anaemia – although he/she would not be able to

---

iii I say Mr but in reality the worm is hermaphroditic – each individual has both male and female sex organs.

produce healthy red blood cells so he or she would develop anaemia just the same and would, unless treated, eventually die – the anaemia would therefore prove to be pernicious.

How do you know if you have a tapeworm lodging with you? Well, in four out of five cases you won't have any symptoms,[21] though some patients report mild symptoms of fatigue, diarrhoea, vomiting, weight loss, constipation and abdominal pain. Sometimes segments of the worm can be seen in faeces, while other indicators are the tapeworm eggs, which can be seen by examining stools. Doctors may sometimes suspect a tapeworm and ask for a stool sample to be analysed. Treatment is by administering Praziquantel which, you'll be pleased to know, is *not* licensed for human use in the UK (though it can be given to 'named patients'), or Niclosamide, which *is* licensed for human use. Both drugs will destroy the parasite, which then exits your body by the normal method.

One person who has experienced living with a fish tapeworm is Helen, from the UK – here's a short account of her experience.

Parasitic infection and vitamin B$_{12}$ deficiency – Helen's story

My first symptoms were sudden nerve pain in one foot, followed by a mini-stroke. Over the next 13 years various and seemingly unconnected aspects of my health declined until I had reached the point where I was expecting to die before much longer. I had unexplained hypertension, breathing difficulties, serious nerve damage in my entire right leg, no bladder or bowel function, almost constant muscle cramps and random infections, allergic reactions and gastro-intestinal upset. During these years I was given a myriad of tests and procedures, some of which confirmed the symptoms but didn't explain the source of them.

I had resigned myself to the fact that I was going to die, but it was then that I came across a possible explanation for all my symptoms – pernicious anaemia. Fortunately, I was able to get my doctor's cooperation but I was found to have a normal B_{12} level. Despite this, and because of my symptoms, my doctor agreed to trial injections and I responded instantly and spectacularly to them. However, I was never able to reduce from that initial aggressive level of treatment and was allowed to remain on it indefinitely.

After about two years I realised the nerve damage was continuing to worsen and by then had accepted I didn't have pernicious anaemia but that B_{12} and folate supplementation were dealing with many of the other symptoms. Four years after starting B_{12}, I had to begin using a bowel irrigation system every few days and it was several months later that I noticed I had passed a six-inch section of tapeworm. The opportunity was lost to have it examined so I wasn't able to access the treatment. However, I was able to find the treatment elsewhere and treated myself successfully. From then on I was able to manage without any B_{12}/folate supplementation.

I had undergone a combined endoscopy/colonoscopy and the parasite wasn't seen since the middle section of intestine is not looked at. Neither did three separate stool tests reveal it despite specifically looking for evidence of the parasite. The only test which gave any indication was a raised eosinophil level. Sadly, my nerve damage is well past the point of recovery and my ongoing problems are now due to the damage sustained over that prolonged period. Perhaps a capsule endoscopy might have revealed the parasite, but this procedure is relatively new and not yet in regular use.

Fish tapeworm isn't the only parasite that causes B_{12} deficiency – and that is why you should think twice before swimming in the dams built by beavers.

Beaver fever

Named after a parasite that is found in the stagnant waters of beaver dams, *Giardia lamblia*, beaver fever is characterised by 'explosive diarrhoea', excessive wind in the form of flatulence, belching that is so foul and sulphuric-tasting that it causes the patient to vomit, pale, foul-smelling greasy stools (steatorrhoea), gastric pain, bloating, nausea, diminished interest in food and sometimes violent vomiting.[22] The scientific name for beaver fever is giardiasis and it's been around for a long time. Recent evidence shows that it was a problem for the crusaders in the 13th century, though it was certainly doing the rounds for hundreds if not thousands of years before that. *Giardia lamblia* is difficult to detect and is frequently misdiagnosed in humans (cats, dogs, sheep, cattle and beavers are also favourites of the parasite), with the diagnosis involving multiple stool examinations which can give false positive indications. And while you may be feeling comfortable that you don't play host to this little beauty of a freeloader you may want to know that about 50% of carriers are asymptomatic in that they carry the parasite but don't (yet) experience any of the symptoms. *Giardia lamblia* lives in the small intestine and enjoys vitamin B_{12} to the extent that it can cause significant B_{12} deficiency[23] and is one of the reasons why you are told to wash your hands thoroughly after using the lavatory, because as well as being transmitted in water the parasite can also be transmitted via a faecal-oral route. There have been recent outbreaks in Oslo and Sydney so it isn't just stagnant backwaters that are prone to infection.

There is controversy surrounding the different medicines used to treat giardiasis because the side effects of the treatment are almost as bad as the symptoms. Animals are treated using a mixture of antibiotics and quarantine, and whilst it is relatively easy to treat cats and dogs, calves can sometimes die. Still, things could be worse – if you were a chinchilla with giardiasis you would definitely die, which is why you have to take care to ensure chinchillas are always given clean, fresh water as they don't respond to medicine. Talking of medicines let's take a look at another, surprising cause of vitamin B_{12} deficiency.

Medicines

There are an enormous number of medicines available to today's doctors and whilst, in years gone by, some of these medicines have proved to have serious and long-lasting side effects, modern medicines are comparatively safe after having undergone rigorous testing and long-term trials before being approved for use. Having said that, most medicines will cause side effects to some degree or other, but these are usually mild. I say mild because there are exceptions and good doctors will make their patients aware of these before prescribing a drug. In addition, as an added precaution to make sure patients are aware of any consequential side effects of a medicine, manufacturers are obliged to include a patient information leaflet with the medicine. These leaflets may list an alarming number of possible side effects which sometimes leads to patients not taking a medicine, but the information is there all the same and reading it is seen as good practice.

It may come as some surprise to you that a wide range of often-prescribed medicines may lead to vitamin B_{12} deficiency. The reason why this happens involves some complex chemistry and we need not go into that in any great detail, but basically, some medicines and their contents are released into body fluids[iv] whilst others interfere with the absorption of vitamin B_{12} in the first place. Either way, these medicines interfere with the metabolism of folate and B_{12}, leading to the patient's store of B_{12} becoming compromised in one way or another, and this could lead eventually to a deficiency in B_{12}.

That some medicines have an impact on patients' B_{12} is not that surprising considering the number of medicines now available – one or two of them would be bound to have a side effect that would affect B_{12}. However, what is truly astonishing is that the medicines that have the biggest impact on B_{12} are not only some of the most commonly prescribed drugs, but also that their effect on patients' B_{12} is rarely, if ever, pointed out by the prescribing physician. For example, one of the medicines that lowers vitamin B_{12} levels is the commonly prescribed contraceptive pill. Now, if you are of a certain gender there is the likelihood that you have, at some time in your life, been prescribed the contraceptive pill. Try to think of when you were first prescribed it – were you warned that it could cause vitamin B_{12} deficiency? The answer is probably not, yet all the time you were enjoying the fruits of the liberal 1960s your B_{12} was being compromised.

Another commonly prescribed medicine that may deplete B_{12} is ibuprofen, used to relieve rheumatic pain. Likewise, colchicine that is used to treat gout; cimetidine and other histamine H2-blockers that are used to treat peptic ulcers; Omeprazole and Lansoprazole – proton pump inhibitors; and some anti-epileptic drugs (phenobarbital, pregabalin, primidone and topiramate).There are also medicines that directly affect the patient's ability to absorb B_{12}, including Metformin – used to treat type 2 diabetes.[24]

All of these common and not so commonly prescribed medicines have the potential to eventually cause B_{12} deficiency and consequently anaemia, though this is not well known, not only among patients but also among medical professionals.

[iv] This is called *haemolysis*, where the red blood cell ruptures and its contents are released into the surrounding plasma.

Thankfully, whilst some of the above do have a substantial effect on B_{12} status (most notably the proton pump inhibitors), most have only a minimal or slight impact and taking a supplement of the vitamin will normally correct any deficiency caused by the medicine. The best course of action if you are worried about the impact your medicine is having on your B_{12} levels is to discuss taking a supplement with your doctor. **You should never stop taking your medicine until you have spoken with your doctor.**

Gastric bypass surgery and ileostomy

As we have seen, the complex process of making healthy red blood cells begins with the production of intrinsic factor (IF) in the stomach and continues when B_{12} + IF is passed into the bloodstream in the part of the small intestine called the ileum. This means that the proper functioning of both the stomach and the ileum is essential.

Gastric bypass surgery involves reducing the stomach by as much as 90% by carefully partitioning it. The result of this is that patients feel 'full' after eating only a small amount of food; it is hoped this will then reduce the amount of food they want to eat and they will lose weight. Obviously partitioning the stomach will compromise the amount of intrinsic factor that is available and consequently the amount of B_{12} that will be absorbed in the bloodstream; consequently, patients are in danger of becoming deficient in B_{12} and should be prescribed oral B_{12} tablets to counteract this.

An ileostomy (surgically producing a new opening in the ileum) is performed when the large intestine (which eventually carries away waste food in the form of faeces) is no longer functioning properly. This could be for a number of reasons, including cancers of the colon or rectum which have had to be removed. The ileum is the final part of the small intestine and in healthy bowels, once the B_{12} has been removed, waste food passes from it into the large intestine.

To create an ileostomy, an incision is made into the bottom of the ileum so that waste products can be collected in an *ostomy pouch* which the patient wears on the side of his or her lower abdomen. An artificial opening is made (called a stoma) to which the bag is attached. This is similar to, though not the same as, the ileocolic resection that was mentioned in the last chapter and, just as in the resection, because part of the ileum has been removed to create the stoma, the patient will subsequently not absorb as much B$_{12}$ as he or she once would have done and so will usually need additional B$_{12}$ in the form of injections or maybe tablets.

Emma's story

I was born April 1962, a normal, home birth with no complications. My parents recall that all was fine with me until 1970, when I developed a nasty sickness and diarrhoea bug that lasted for over a week and resulted in me being severely dehydrated and hospitalised for a further week. Whilst in hospital my parents were told I had gastric enteritis and strep throat.

Following this illness I started to get frequent urgent bouts of diarrhoea and crampy abdominal pains after eating many foods that had previously caused me no problems; this would continue throughout my life. These bouts made me anxious about going out and stopped me from going to play at other children's houses where I would feel worried that diarrhoea might 'strike' and where the mothers of my friends would frequently say how 'fussy' I was about food. As a result, I stuck with my best friend whose family understood my situation.

I was so tired throughout my childhood and teenage years. My Mum remembers how I would say I was going to play in my room and put a 'Do not Disturb' sign on the door and she would then find me asleep in bed with my toys untouched. I would ask to go to bed frequently and I would always be there between 8 pm and 9pm at the latest; this continued even after I left school. I often wondered why I didn't have the energy that others my age seemed to have, but sleep was always my priority because without it I felt awful. In 1976, aged 14, I developed a bout of tonsillitis that lasted two months and would not respond to antibiotics. I became allergic to several antibiotics during this time and ended up having twice-daily injections of antibiotics as my throat was almost closed. The doctors suggested that I was also suffering from glandular fever and that the tonsillitis was a secondary bacterial infection.

The tiredness and sudden bouts of diarrhoea continued and I tried to sleep as much as possible. I visited my GP on several occasions to complain of my tiredness and was always told it was because I was a teenager, or hormonal, but no further investigations were done.

In 1984 I was hospitalised with a kidney infection, and went into anaphylactic shock during a scan using IV iodine whilst the doctors looked for kidney stones. (I don't think they found any; as I had seizures and became unconscious I wasn't aware of much!)

By 1984 I was being seen at Addenbrooke's Hospital in Cambridge for suspected food intolerance because of my continuing bouts of diarrhoea and the constant fatigue. I was put on a strict exclusion diet, but although I felt a little better the problems continued.

In 1988 I had my first son delivered by emergency caesarean section six weeks early due to abruption of the placenta. In 1989 I had a biopsy taken for an abnormal smear; this caused a haemorrhage several days later and I was hospitalised and given a plasma transfusion because I had lost so much blood. In June 1990, I had appendicitis and had my appendix removed.

The above is background information may or may not be relevant but my feeling is that I may have had pernicious anaemia from childhood, although I obviously can't prove that.

My story (proper) starts in November 1990 when I had my terminal ileum surgically removed following peritonitis caused by adhesions from the appendix removal six months previously. The last 45 centimetres of my terminal ileum was removed and I remained in hospital for two weeks to recover. I became doubly incontinent which is horrible for anyone but very tricky as a 28-year-old with a toddler to care for. For six months I remained that way, losing weight, not able to go out and unable to control the diarrhoea.

After six months of trying various medications that did not work the gastroenterologist suggested trying Questran which was given to patients to reduce cholesterol but had the side effect of causing constipation. Thankfully this helped a lot and I remained on this treatment for nearly 25 years.

The consultant did not mention B$_{12}$ or that I should be having injections following my surgery; he did say I'd lost the most useful bit of my gut and that the diarrhoea might take a while to settle. Then I was discharged and told to get on with my life, which I did although the diarrhoea never did settle without the Questran.

In 1996 I became pregnant with my second son, after trying for four years and being told I would be unable to conceive again naturally due, the doctors said, to the amount of abdominal surgery I had had and the adhesion problem.

My son was born at 32 weeks by emergency caesarean section, this time due to the placenta breaking up causing bleeding and foetal distress. He was born with an enlarged liver and his lungs collapsed. He stayed in intensive care and then high dependency care for two months until he was able to leave hospital.

My tiredness became worse, the diarrhoea remained and I began to suffer from frequent headaches. I was prescribed antidepressants.

During my second pregnancy I had developed acne and then later that year I was diagnosed with rosacea. I had a negative blood test for possible lupus. I tried to get on with things and slept during the afternoons whenever I could in order to be functional in the evenings.

In 1999 I was back at the GP's feeling exhausted and was told that a blood test showed neutropenia [white blood cell deficiency] but the GP said this was not a concern.

In 2002, aged 40, I had a third son, again delivered by

emergency caesarean section, this time at 36 weeks as a scan showed no amniotic fluid around baby.

My husband and I managed to cope but the tiredness was overwhelming. I started bumping into door frames and became clumsy, putting cups and plates down and missing the work tops; I became forgetful and I suffered from constant headaches. I would get trembling hands and legs and would grab something to eat and sit until the feeling passed. Another trip to the GP for blood tests showed neutropenia again and he suggested the trembling was probably hypoglycaemia and that I should eat more breakfast or carry a snack at all times.

In 2005, I was referred to a neurologist as I was still shoulder-bumping door frames and had fallen over backwards twice whilst carrying my toddler son. The neurologist listened to my account of my symptoms and examined me. I had very brisk reflexes and he agreed that it seemed strange, but when my brain scan came back normal he said not to worry about the symptoms and carry on as normal.

In July 2006 I saw a locum GP and once again listed my symptoms, including the extreme tiredness. She asked me when I had had my last B$_{12}$ injection and I told her I had never had one. She seemed surprised and told me they would give me three-monthly injections and that I would soon be feeling better. She didn't elaborate but I went away relieved that something as simple as an injection was going to make me better.

I had my first injection but didn't notice any difference in my symptoms. I continued to have the injections every three to six months over the next three years but didn't feel much better.

In 2007 I developed a severe allergy to the sun and was told I had polymorphic light eruption.

At the beginning of 2010 I went for my B_{12} injection and I was told that they were going to take a blood test to see if I still needed the B_{12}; the results came back and I was told I no longer needed injections. I didn't argue; I didn't know any better then and as I hadn't had a miraculous recovery from my symptoms when I was having them I accepted the situation.

In 2013, along with the tiredness and headaches, I had developed a burning sensation along the outside of my right foot. In addition, my hair was breaking and falling out and I was constantly yawning while walking the dog. I had developed eczema on my hand and by now my vision was blurry. My GP arranged blood tests and said my iron levels were low and put me on iron supplements.

By 2014 I had pins and needles in my feet, hands and around my mouth, intermittent burning feelings in my feet, and loss of hot/cold sensations in my feet and hands. I revisited my GP. She mentioned that we should see what the blood tests said but she might consider sending me to a rheumatologist if the symptoms continued. I'm pretty sure she thought I was a hypochondriac and I could sense her frustration so I decided to see a rheumatologist privately as I was getting worse week by week. The pins and needles in my feet had now travelled up to the top of both my legs and up from my hands as far as my elbows.

My legs started giving way in August 2014, just before my first appointment with the rheumatologist who examined me, and when I couldn't feel the pin prick test on my legs or arms she suggested I have some nerve conduction studies and that I should see a neurologist. She also noticed from a previous blood test that my cortisol levels were low and suggested a synacthen test to rule out Addison's disease. The nerve conduction studies showed a small fibre peripheral neuropathy while the synacthen test was normal.

The rheumatologist wrote to the neurologist with her findings and mentioned that she had heard B$_{12}$ deficiency could cause my symptoms and that she would welcome his thoughts on that. By the time I saw the neurologist my legs had given way on several more occasions. I had all my previous symptoms plus tinnitus in my right ear, jerking legs when resting, frequent need to urinate, and confusion; I even said to my husband I thought I might have dementia. The neurologist was the same person I had seen nine years before; he felt there couldn't be too much wrong with me, said he didn't know much about B$_{12}$ but he would arrange a brain scan again.

The brain scan came back normal and he suggested I try taking sodium valproate (an anti-epileptic drug) to try to control the headaches. I felt he had missed the point totally and have not followed his suggestion in this case.

In desperation I started trawling the internet and using symptom checker websites. They all said the same thing

– B_{12} deficiency, and that permanent nerve damage could result if left untreated. I checked out the $B_{12}D$ website and found a link to Pernicious Anaemia Society. I ordered both Martyn's books and the *Could it be B_{12}?* book from Amazon and devoured them! Everything I was reading described me. I was excited to have found something that made sense and at the same time I was scared that I had discovered it too late.

I returned to my surgery to see a locum GP with my husband in tow for support and with material from PA Society website about treatment. Luckily, she read the information and agreed that I should have B_{12} injections again and that I could have them every other day as long as I agreed to see a haematologist who could decide what to do next. So on 28th October 2014 I started the injections. Once again I didn't feel much difference but the fuzziness in my head seemed to improve a little so I was hopeful.

Next I went to see a haematologist and she confirmed that due to my ileal surgery I should have been having B_{12} injections since 1990 and that my symptoms were those of B_{12} deficiency. She said to continue the injections until there was no further improvement. While there, I had a blood test for intrinsic factor antibodies, which came back negative, and a methylmalonic acid test on a urine sample, which came back normal. I had had an injection the day before, which probably affected the results.

I continued to have the injections three times a week until my GP told me they had to stop because the auditors had questioned it; it was against protocol and I was taking up too much of the nurse's time! I contacted the haematologist who said that as I didn't seem to be improving much I should continue the B$_{12}$ jabs monthly. This was when I decided that I would self-inject using methylcobalamin that I obtained from a reliable source.

I continued to inject daily for several weeks but with no change in symptoms and I saw a private doctor who suggested an intravenous infusion of B$_{12}$. I had that but, combined with a strict detox diet for a month, there was no change in my symptoms.

So, here I am – 53 years old and with the following issues: continually feeling exhausted; pins and needles in my legs, hands and around my mouth; legs that give way three times a week on average; and days when I find it hard to speak and can't find the words or think what things are called. Since 2004 I have had a persistent cough, the cause of which has never been found despite several investigations. I have difficulty swallowing when eating which has been put down to weak muscles in my oesophagus though no reason has been given as to why they should be weak. I have a continual burning feeling in my right foot, tinnitus in my right ear, frequent headaches and hazy vision (like when you go back to watching normal television after watching in HD). In 2014 I developed vitiligo, my hair is falling out, I have brittle nails, rosacea, polymorphic light eruptions and eczema on my hand and have now developed wheat and lactose sensitivity. All of this means that I sometimes get depressed. Apart from all of the above, I'm fine! Seriously though, I know it's not the end of the world and there are plenty worse things that people have, but it does make life with a family of three boys, the youngest on the autistic spectrum, tough.

I have adapted my life over the years to accommodate my problems and have been sleeping every afternoon over the past 10 years just to try to keep going and be able to function and get meals and put children to bed etcetera in the evening. I don't know what to do now; I feel I have exhausted all avenues and have used up money trying to get a diagnosis and treatment to no avail.

Author's comment: There are two things to note here. Firstly, there are patients who have had their ileum removed but have not been prescribed vitamin B_{12} to compensate for not subsequently being able to absorb the vitamin from food. Maybe Emma's case is unusual, an oversight that shouldn't have happened; on the other hand, I have heard of several cases where the prescription has been stopped because a routine test to determine the patient's B_{12} status showed high levels of the vitamin in his or her blood. If *you* know of somebody who has undergone an ileostomy it might be worth checking that he/she is receiving regular replacement B_{12} injections; these should be given for life and regardless of the results of any serum B_{12} test. Secondly, it demonstrates that even with enormous amounts of replacement B_{12} patients don't always see their symptoms relieved. Could this be because of the time taken to address any deficiency? Is there a correlation between the time taken to identify and treat any B_{12} deficiency and the persistence of the symptoms of that deficiency? It's an interesting question but one that has not been addressed by anyone.

Nitrous oxide (N_2O) – 'laughing gas'

Every year the UK's Home Office publishes a survey of drug use in the past year in the UK.[25] Overall, drug use in the UK is declining, though the use of cocaine bucks this trend and is on the increase. In 2012/13 cannabis was the most commonly used drug, with 6.4% of adults aged 16 to 59 using it in the previous year, while powder cocaine came second, with 1.9% of adults using it in the previous year. In third place was ecstasy, with 1.3% of the population having used it in the previous year.

In 2013 for the first time the UK's Home Office included in the results of its annual survey two new 'legal highs' – the plant Salvia, which is a member of the sage family, and nitrous oxide.

Altogether 0.5% of adults aged 16 to 59 had taken Salvia in the previous year and presumably enjoyed the experience – it causes the user to revisit past memories, experience sensations of motion or being pulled or twisted by forces, alters vision so the user thinks he or she is looking through a membrane or film, and causes uncontrollable laughter. Unless it is used in very high quantities there are no lasting side effects, and no effect on levels of B_{12}. The same cannot be said for nitrous oxide.

Nitrous oxide: Altogether 2.3% of adults aged 16 to 59 had taken nitrous oxide in the previous year, which makes it (fanfare please) the second most used recreational drug after cannabis in 2012/13 – it had more users than cocaine. Nitrous oxide causes the user to laugh – hence its more common name 'laughing gas' – and it has one lasting side effect: it 'inactivates' vitamin B_{12}. Inactive B_{12} cannot play its vital part in methionine synthase, which is needed to make methylcobalamin available. (It does this by oxidising the cobalt I [Co+] form of cobalamin [vitamin B_{12}] to Co3+ and the resulting oxidised cobalt cation prevents cobalamin [vitamin B_{12}] acting as a coenzyme for methionine synthase.) The chemistry need not concern us but here's what a paper from 2008 has to say about nitrous oxide and B_{12}:

> Certain patient groups may be particularly susceptible to reduced methionine synthase activity, including those deficient in cobalamin, such as patients with pernicious anemia or ileal disease, alcoholics, the elderly, and the malnourished.[26]

And if the vitamin B_{12} has been inactivated by the nitrous oxide, the paper goes on to say: '...simultaneous inactivation of vitamin B_{12} may produce nitrous oxide's neurotoxic effects.' The 'neurotoxic effects' are neurological damage. And there's more:

> Neurologic injury has also been noted after a routine nitrous oxide-based anesthetic in patients with cobalamin deficiency, such as those with pernicious anemia, although the injury did not become apparent for many weeks.

Another paper from 2013 also warns of the effects of the recreational use of N_2O:

> N_2O abuse may induce vitamin B_{12} deficiency, leading to hyperpigmentation of the skin, hair changes, megaloblastic anemia, pancytopenia, sub-acute combined degeneration, depression, psychosis, and a possible increased risk of myocardial infarction and stroke.[27]

So the message is, even if you are tempted to join the party and sniff a lungful of N_2O, be aware that the effects of your B_{12} deficiency, even if it is not caused by pernicious anaemia, will be made much worse. Nitrous oxide is widely available at music festivals and nightclubs where it is sold by the balloon-full. Those who prefer to laugh their heads off in the comfort of their own homes can purchase equipment from the internet or cookshops to fill balloons themselves. (This 'equipment' consists of 'whippets' which are canisters made for dispensing whipped cream, which contain a small bulb of pressurised nitrous oxide intended to whip cream as it is forced out. If the cream is left out, the gas can be released and captured in a balloon over the nozzle. A quick search of YouTube shows many videos of young people sucking in balloons of nitrous oxide and having a great laugh, but be careful. It is not as carefree an activity as it appears.)

Before we leave nitrous oxide as a cause of B$_{12}$ deficiency there's something else you should know – if you work in an operating theatre or dental surgery that uses nitrous oxide you could be adversely affected whether you have pernicious anaemia or not: 'Occupational exposure to high levels of nitrous oxide may adversely affect a woman's ability to become pregnant.[28]

However, another paper challenges this and insists that this is only the case if the person is also deficient in B$_{12}$:

> Occupational N$_2$O exposure of medical and dental
> personnel during its use as an analgesic is not likely to produce adverse reproductive outcomes except in B$_{12}$-deficient
> individuals or in those routinely exposed to
> high N$_2$O levels.[29]

Note that another common medical use of N$_2$O is in 'gas and air' used during childbirth and by paramedics.

From the above it can be seen there are several causes of B$_{12}$ deficiency, but what exactly is deemed to be 'deficiency'? In the next chapter I address the problems of how we measure the B$_{12}$ status of the population, or rather, how we don't measure it accurately. And this is where we start to make some remarkable discoveries.

References

1   Hunt A, Harrington D, Robinson S. Vitamin B12 deficiency. *British Medical Journal* 2014; 349: 5226.

2   Office for National Statistics. *2011 Census: Usual resident population by five-year age group and sex, local authorities in the United Kingdom.* http://www.ons.gov.uk/ons/guide-method/census/2011/index.html (Accessed 7 January 2012).

3   US Census Bureau. *Census 2000 Summary File 1 and 2010 Census Summary File 1.* http://www.census.gov/prod/cen2010/briefs/c2010br-03.pdf (Accessed 7 January 2015).

4   Ibid 3.

5   Wikipedia. *Demography of India.* https://en.wikipedia.org/wiki/Demographics_of_India (Accessed 7 January 2015).

6   Stabler S, Allen R. Vitamin B12 deficiency as a worldwide problem. *Annual Review of Nutrition* 2004; 24:299–326.

7   Andres E, Serraj K. Optimal management of pernicious anemia. *Journal of Blood Medicine* 2012; 3:97–103..

8   Hooper M, Hudson P, Porter F, McCaddon A. Patient journeys: the diagnosis and treatment of pernicious anaemia. *British Journal of Nursing* 2014; 23(7):16-21.

9   Pawlak R, Lester SE, Babatunde T. The prevalence of cobalamin deficiency among vegetarians assessed by serum vitamin B12: a review of literature. *European Journal of Clinical Nutrition* 2014; 68:541-548. doi: 10.1038/ejcn.2014.46

10   Foster R, Lunn J. 40th Anniversary briefing paper: food availability and our changing diet. *Nutrition Bulletin* 2007; 32:187–249.

11   www.waterfootprint.org/ http://waterfootprint.org/media/downloads/Hoekstra-2008-WaterfootprintFood.pdf (Accessed 9 December 2014).

12   Van Huis A, Van Itterbeek J, Klunder H, Mertens E, Halloran A, Muir G, Vantomme P. *Edible insects: future prospects for food and feed security.* FAO Forestry Paper 171. Rome: FAO; 2013.

13 Finke MD. Nutrient Content of Insects. In: *Encyclopedia of Entomology* Netherlands: Springer; 2004: 2623-2646. http://www. organicvaluerecovery.com/studies/studies_nutrient_content_of_ insects.htm (Accessed 6 December 2014).

14 Watanabe F, Yabuta Y, Bito T, Teng F. Vitamin B12-containing plant food sources for vegetarians. Nutrients 2014; 6, 1861–1873. (Accessed 6 December 2014).

15 Vogiatzoglou AV, Smith AD, Nurk E, Berstad P, Drevon CA, Ueland PM, Vollset SE, Tell GS, Refsum H. Dietary sources of vitamin B-12 and their association with plasma vitamin B-12 concentrations in the general population: the Hordland Homocysteine Study 1–3. *American Journal of Clinical Nutrition* 2009; 89(4):1078–1087.

16 Kusters JG, van Vliet AH, Kuipers EJ. Pathogenesis of Helicobacter pylori Infection. *Clinical Microbiology Reviews* 2006; 19(3):449–490.

17 Pounder RE, Ng D. The prevalence of Helicobacter pylori infection in different countries. *Alimentary Pharmacology and Therapeutics* 1995; 9(Suppl 2):33–39.

18 UN Food and Agriculture Organisation and World Health Organisation. Human Vitamin and Mineral Requirements. Rome; FAO/WHO; 2001. http://www.fao.org/docrep/004/y2809e/ y2809e0b.htm (Accessed 20 April 2015).,

19 Ibid (ref 17).

20 Von Bonsdorff B, Gordin R. Castle's test (with vitamin B12 and normal gastric juice) in the ileum in patients with genuine and patients with tapeworm pernicious anaemia. *Acta Medica Scandinavica* 1980; 208(3):193–197.

21 Scholz T, Garcia HH, Kuchta R, Wicht B. Update on the human broad tapeworm (genus Diphyllobothrium), including clinical relevance. *Clinical Microbiology Reviews* 2009; 22(1):146–160.

22 Huang DB, White AC. An updated review on Cryptosporidium and Giardia. *Gastroenterology Clinics of North America*. 2006; 35 (2):291–314, viii.

23 Cordingley FT, Crawford GP. Giardia infection causes vitamin B12 deficiency. *Australian and New Zealand Journal of Medicine* 1986; 16(1):78–79.

24 David SH, Bell MD. Metformin-induced vitamin B12 deficiency presenting as a peripheral neuropathy. *Southern Medical Journal* 2010; 103(3):265–267.

25 Office for National Statistics. *Drug Misuse: Findings from the 2012 to 2013 Crime Survey for England and Wales.* https://www.gov.uk/government/publications/drug-misuse-findings-from-the-2012-to-2013-csew/drug-misuse-findings-from-the-2012-to-2013-crime-survey-for-england-and-wales (Accessed 20 August 2014).

26 Sanders RD, Weimann J, Maze M. Biologic effects of nitrous oxide: a mechanistic and toxicologic review. *Anesthesiology* 2008; 109:707–722.

27 Tsung-Ta C, Chih-Tsung H, Wei-Ming W, Jiunn-Tay L, Fu-Chi Y. Recreational nitrous oxide abuse-induced vitamin B12 deficiency in a patient presenting with hyperpigmentation of the skin. *Case Reports in Dermatology* 2013; 5:186–191.

28 Roland AS Baird DD, Weinberg CR, Shore DL, Shy CM, Wilcox AJ. Reduced fertility among women employed as dental assistants exposed to high levels of nitrous oxide. *New England Journal of Medicine* 1992; 327:993–997.

29 Louis-Ferdinand RT. Myelotoxic, neurotoxic and reproductive adverse effects of nitrous oxide. *Adverse Drug Reactions Toxicology Review* 1994; 13(4):193–206.

Chapter 3

Problems in diagnosing vitamin B12 deficiency

For some years there has been much anecdotal evidence that there are problems with the diagnosis of vitamin B$_{12}$ deficiency. The recent survey of members of the Pernicious Anaemia Society mentioned in the Introduction (page xv) demonstrates quite clearly that this is the case: there is a problem with patients who are deficient in vitamin B$_{12}$ receiving a timely and accurate explanation for their symptoms. The results of the survey reflect the experiences of patients posting their experiences of misdiagnosis and wrong diagnosis on a wide variety of social media. In that sense the survey can be seen as providing a numeric value for the widespread anecdotal evidence that is available on the internet. Let's take a look at some of the figures from the survey:[i]

- 304 individuals experienced symptoms of the disorder for up to a year before a diagnosis of pernicious anaemia was made
- some had to wait up two years (193), five years (173), 10 years (40) or more

[i] These figures are taken from a survey of 889 members of the Pernicious Anaemia Society who live in the UK – 1184 members completed the survey but it was decided to concentrate solely on UK members because different countries have different treatment regimens which would have made the data about treatment meaningless.

- 127 individuals experienced symptoms for more than 10 years prior to receiving their diagnosis.

Now, before you reach for your calculator I've worked out the percentages for you:

- 34% of patients waited 'up to a year' for a diagnosis, which I suppose is because the symptoms are so vague and wide-ranging
- more worrying is that 21% waited between one and two years for an accurate diagnosis and 19% of patients waited between two and five years to be diagnosed; add those two figures together and 40% of patients waited between one and five years to be accurately diagnosed
- a staggering 14% had to wait over 10 years for a diagnosis; that's worth saying again: 14% waited *over* 10 years for an accurate diagnosis.

These statistics take on a whole new meaning when you consider that left undiagnosed a B$_{12}$ deficiency can and does lead to severe and irreversible nerve damage. There's obviously a problem with the way in which B$_{12}$ deficiency is identified, and whether that deficiency is caused by pernicious anaemia. Actually, there isn't just one problem but rather a series of problems that I will explore in this chapter. I will do so by tackling each barrier to an early diagnosis one by one.

Problem 1: The symptoms

There are four main issues with the symptoms of B$_{12}$ deficiency leading to a late diagnosis.

Symptoms take a long time to develop

Firstly, the symptoms themselves are insidious in that they often take many years to manifest themselves to the extent that the patient becomes fully aware of them. A little breathlessness is often attributed to a little extra exertion; a slight memory loss is seen as age-related; the tiredness is often put down to a busy modern lifestyle. These three classic symptoms are sure signs of a possible B_{12} deficiency, but they are often ignored by the patient and attributed to normal living. By the time they become noticeable and start to have an impact on the patient's everyday life, the vitamin deficiency may have been present for many years. The Pernicious Anaemia Society's new range of posters address this issue, urging patients to talk to their doctor about their symptoms and to not ignore them or attribute them to something else. This little chat with their GP then brings us nicely onto the second issue – the symptoms of B_{12} deficiency are very broad and vague.

Symptoms can be broad and vague

Take a look at the list of symptoms that are indicators of B_{12} deficiency in Appendix 2. You will begin to appreciate how the deficiency affects almost all aspects of human health and, perhaps more importantly, how the symptoms relate to different medical disciplines, such as urology, psychiatry, gastroenterology, endocrinology, paediatrics and child health, obstetrics and gynaecology. All these disciplines can become involved in the symptoms of B_{12} deficiency, demonstrating the wide-ranging nature of the indicators of a deficiency in the vitamin. This wide range of symptoms often means that the patient is embarrassed to talk about his or her symptoms because of the concern that he or she might be considered a hypochondriac and a 'moaner'. I can vouch that when people with pernicious anaemia get together with other sufferers they are relieved to discover that other patients also suffer a wide range of symptoms, often swapping a long list of their experiences with others and realising with great relief that they aren't imagining their indicators of B_{12} deficiency even after treatment has begun (more of this later – see page 129).

The survey demonstrates that often sufferers had attributed these broad symptoms to lifestyle or advancing age. This issue is difficult to address. It means that primary care physicians need to be made aware of how wide-ranging the symptoms are, and this leads us to the third problem with the symptoms – they are associated with other medical conditions and not solely with pernicious anaemia.

Symptoms are associated with other diseases

Let's take the most common symptom of pernicious anaemia – tiredness. A quick look at the UK's *NHS Choices* website gives 10 medical reasons why a person becomes tired. These include the following:

- coeliac disease (especially if accompanied by diarrhoea, anaemia and weight loss)
- anaemia – especially if you have heavy periods – specifically iron-deficiency anaemia
- sleep apnoea
- underactive thyroid
- diabetes
- glandular fever
- depression
- restless legs
- anxiety.

It's not surprising that this single most common symptom leads doctors to suspect something other than pernicious anaemia. According to our survey, 44% of respondents were originally told their symptoms were due to a condition other than pernicious anaemia, with 37% of patients originally diagnosed as suffering from some of the above: 2% were originally told they had coeliac disease, 5% iron deficiency, 4% underactive thyroid, 16% anxiety and another 5% chronic fatigue syndrome. These are not co-existing conditions but initial misdiagnoses based on just one symptom of pernicious anaemia – tiredness.

Now, if you look at the vast range of other symptoms associated with pernicious anaemia then it is easy to see how doctors are often led towards some other diagnosis – I was originally told I had multiple sclerosis, for example, before being told the correct reason for my nerve damage.

Symptoms vary in their severity

The fourth issue with the symptoms of B_{12} deficiency relates to the degree to which the patient experiences the symptoms, because not only are the symptoms wide and varied but also they manifest themselves to varying degrees; some patients will experience chronic, uncontrollable diarrhoea while others will only have loose motions. Some patients will have mood swings that are so sudden and extreme that their everyday work is compromised, to the extent that disciplinary procedures are started against them, while others may experience only a general moroseness that soon disappears. Some patients may experience the neurological problems to the extent that they cannot walk while others may have occasional pins and needles and a little numbness in their feet.

There are two further problems here. Firstly, patients may ignore any subtle manifestation of their symptoms, attributing them to various causes and not mentioning them to their doctor – but they do so at their peril because subtle experiences have a habit of developing into serious and life-changing symptoms that sometimes are impossible to reverse. Secondly, patients may mention these subtle indicators of there being something 'not right', but the physician may attribute them to something else – lifestyle, change of job or career etc. It's surprising how many people are told that any pins and needles or numbness in their feet is probably due to their footwear.

The lesson here is for patients to be thoroughly honest with their GP and to tell him or her *all* of their symptoms no matter how bizarre or subtle they may be. Of course, that could mean that the patient reels off a long list that includes emotional as well as physical, psychiatric and neurological manifestations, and this might mean the GP is left bewildered and the patient feeling a little silly. What needs to be done is to make GPs aware of this vast range of possible symptoms of B_{12} deficiency; this is why the new website of the Pernicious Anaemia Society has a special section for medical professionals that gives a formidable list of indicators of the disease.

To sum up, there is a whole range of problems with the symptoms of vitamin B_{12} deficiency/pernicious anaemia – they are broad, often subtle, regularly associated with other diseases, vary in their intensity and patients may be reluctant to discuss them with their doctors.

Problem 2: Doctors don't look for B₁₂ deficiency

A few years ago I was interviewed for a weekly health programme broadcast by the BBC. The presenter was also a practising GP who was interested in the Pernicious Anaemia Society's views that the current practice of providing a replacement therapy injection to patients with pernicious anaemia every three months in the UK was hopelessly inadequate for some, though not all, patients. A week or two after the interview, the presenter emailed to tell me that during the week following the interview he had diagnosed two people as having pernicious anaemia, adding that 'It's surprising what you find when you look for it.' That brings us nicely to the second problem with diagnosing vitamin B_{12} deficiency – doctors don't always look for it.

When patients visit their doctor with a few, or many, of the symptoms associated with B_{12} deficiency, there is no guarantee that the physician will automatically test for low B_{12}. If he or she does decide to investigate further, he/she will probably only request a full blood count initially.[ii] The full blood count will look for the large red blood cells which are an indicator of low B_{12}. Not all doctors routinely request a serum B_{12} test at the same time. Whether your physician checks your B_{12} using the serum test seems to depend on where you live. Now's the time to take a look at the remarkable set of maps in the *NHS Atlas of Variation in Diagnostic Services*, mentioned in the Introduction[iii] (see Figures 3.1–3.4).

The maps show the number of serum B_{12} tests ordered per 1000 patients. They reveal that you are five times more likely to have your B_{12} levels tested in some parts of England than in others. Another way of looking at it is that you are five times *less* likely to have your B_{12} tested in some areas than others.

Why is this? Well, the *Atlas* states that it could be because some doctors will not ask for the specific serum B_{12} test if there are no 'haematological indices' – that is, that unless the patient's full blood count shows some enlarged red blood cells, the doctors will not order the B_{12} test (more of this below – page 78). This is what the *Atlas* says:

> The degree of variation observed in vitamin B_{12} testing
> appears to be greater than can be explained by differences
> in the prevalence of the conditions or deficiencies for which
> vitamin B_{12} tests are used. Part of the variation may relate to
> differences in local protocols with respect to when vitamin
> B_{12} assays are undertaken, for example, some may stipulate
> only when haematological indices indicate possible megalo-
> blastic change. It is important to be aware that neurological
> disorders related to vitamin B_{12} deficiency may occur in the
> absence of any haematological change.

[ii] See Appendix 3 for a full list of tests that form the full blood count.
[iii] These maps only cover England. No such maps exist for the other parts of the UK or, as far as I'm aware, anywhere else in the world.

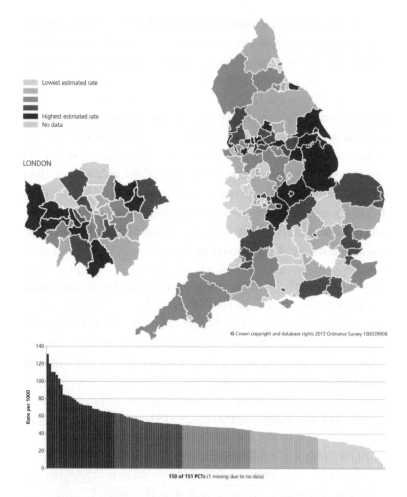

Figure 3.1 Estimated annual rate of use for vitamin B_{12} tests ordered by GP per practice population by PCT. (From Public Health England, *The NHS Atlas of Variation in Diagnostic Services* RightCare NHS; 2013, with permission.)

Given that vitamin B_{12} deficiency is so widespread, shouldn't the serum B_{12} test be routinely carried out as part of the full blood count? If it was, then it would mean that the regional variations would not be so great or maybe would disappear altogether. However, this

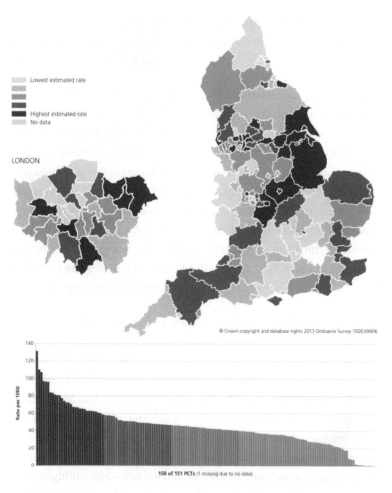

Figure 3.2 Estimated annual rate of use for serum folate tests ordered by GP per practice population by PCT. (From Public Health England, *The NHS Atlas of Variation in Diagnostic Services* RightCare NHS; 2013, with permission.)

means that doctors would rely on the serum B_{12} test to determine any deficiency in B_{12}, but as we shall see next, there are problems with the test itself.

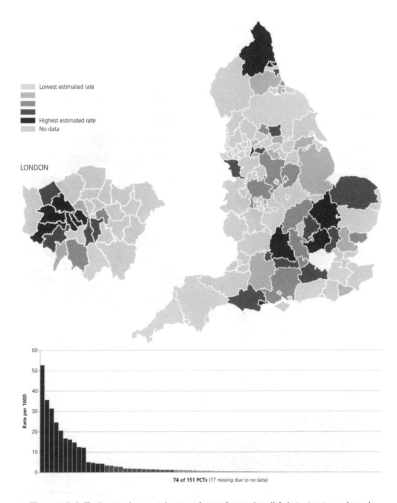

Figure 3.3 Estimated annual rate of use for red cell folate tests ordered by GP per practice population by PCT. (From Public Health England, *The NHS Atlas of Variation in Diagnostic Services* RightCare NHS; 2013, with permission.)

Problem 3: Blood count tests do not find enlarged red blood cells

Let's imagine that the patient has visited his or her GP and told him or her all of the symptoms being experienced. The GP will suspect

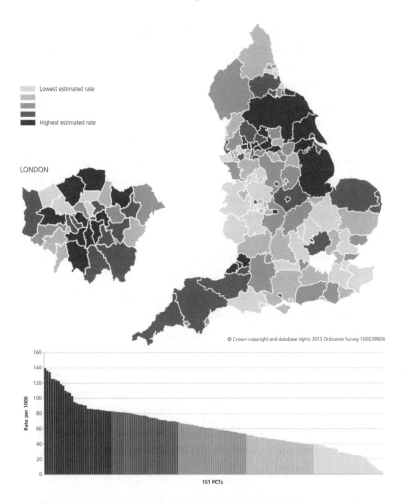

Figure 3.4 Estimated annual rate of use for ferritin tests ordered by GP per practice population by PCT. (From Public Health England, *The NHS Atlas of Variation in Diagnostic Services* RightCare NHS; 2013, with permission.)

vitamin B_{12} deficiency and will order a full blood count. The full blood count will not routinely assess the patient's B_{12} status but will look for signs of macrocytosis (enlarged red blood cells)[iv] that could

---

[iv] Macrocytosis is the name given by doctors to enlarged red blood cells.

be an indicator of B$_{12}$ deficiency, but actually occur only in around 60% of cases. Here are some extracts from the relevant research.

- 'Low serum cobalamin levels in the absence of megaloblastic anemia is also encountered. In a study of 70 consecutive patients with pernicious anemia, only 45 (64%) had very low cobalamin levels (i.e. under 100 pg/ml). Anemia was absent in 13 (19%) and macrocytosis was absent in 23 (33%).'[1]
- 'Among 141 consecutive patients with neuro-psychiatric abnormalities due to cobalamin deficiency, we found that 40 (28%) had no anemia or macrocytosis.'[2]
- 'The absence of a raised MCV[v] cannot be used to exclude the need for cobalamin testing since neurological impairment occurs with a normal MCV in 25% of cases.'[3]
- 'The proscription that cobalamin deficiency should not be diagnosed unless megaloblastic changes are found is akin to requiring jaundice to diagnose liver disease.'[4]

So what this means is that, even if the patient's doctor suspects that the patient's symptoms could be due to low B$_{12}$, unless he or she requests a stand-alone serum B$_{12}$ test, the trusted indicator of possible deficiency – enlarged red blood cells – will not necessarily be present, and consequently the patient will be told that he or she does not have a B$_{12}$ deficiency when in fact he or she may very well do so:

> However, abnormal haemoglobin and erythrocyte mean cell volume values support suspected pernicious anaemia, but normal levels do not rule out the presence of vitamin B$_{12}$ deficiency, leading to a high risk of clinical error. In conclusion, our experience further supports the fact that when the diagnosis of B$_{12}$ deficiency is suspected on the basis of clinical findings and additional tests, supplementation treat-

[v] MCV = Mean corpuscular volume or mean cell volume – they mean the same thing – the size of the red blood cell.

ment should be administered even if the assayed level of the vitamin is not low and, if possible, an assay from another manufacturer is recommended.[5]

There is an additional problem relating to enlarged red blood cells and that centres around vitamin B_9 – our old friend folate (see page 12).

Folic acid fortification

As I mentioned briefly in Chapter 1, there is another issue regarding macrocytosis as an indicator of B_{12} deficiency – taking folic acid supplements can mask this sign of a possible B_{12} deficiency as folic acid stops red blood cells from becoming enlarged. A wide range of foodstuffs are now fortified with folic acid, including all flour in the USA and Canada. The UK is still debating whether or not to go ahead with fortification of flour and there is compelling evidence to do so as it drastically reduces the number of babies born with neural tube defects every year. One study found that:

> The overall prevalence of neural-tube defects at birth
> decreased from 1.58 per 1000 births before fortification to
> 0.86 per 1000 births during the full-fortification period, a
> 46% reduction.[6]

This is why pregnant mothers in the UK are routinely prescribed folic acid during the first part of their pregnancy – it's to ensure that if the mother is deficient in folate then that deficiency is corrected in order to allow the foetus to develop properly. And the reason why this correction takes place is because folate deficiency is quite common in the UK. A recent report[7] reveals that many children in the UK lack adequate levels of folate as defined by the World Health Organisation (WHO):

In children, 2.6% of those aged four to 10 years, 16.9 %
of boys aged 11 to 18 years and 21.8% of girls aged 11 to
18 years had a serum total folate concentration below the
WHO threshold indicating biochemical folate deficiency (10
nmol/l).[7]

That means that in the UK as a whole, over a fifth of teenage girls
are deficient in folate, and the figures aren't much better for adults:

The proportion of adults who had a serum total folate
concentration below the WHO threshold indicating biochemical folate deficiency (10 nmol/l) was 15.5% for men
aged 19 to 64 years, 13.9% for women aged 19 to 64 years,
8.5% for men aged 65 years and over and 12.4% for women
aged 65 years and over.[7]

In other words, nearly 14% of women of child-bearing age in the
UK are deficient in folate, meaning their babies are at risk of spina
bifida or worse unless they receive supplementation. How best to
achieve this supplementation is an as yet unanswered question, but
an important one given there are risks in supplementing the rest of
the population.

Even though there is the risk that fortifying flour with folic acid
could lead to further delays in patients being diagnosed with B$_{12}$
deficiency, the Pernicious Anaemia Society isn't against folic acid
fortification per se, but rather we want a system of regular screening
of B$_{12}$ status in patients to be introduced with a more accurate and
less troublesome assay before this goes ahead. The Society is also
concerned about the possible imbalance that might be caused after
fortification between folate and B$_{12}$ status that can lead to cognitive
impairment in people with low B$_{12}$ status (see Chapter 1, page 15).

All of the above issues centre around enlarged red blood cells as an
indicator of B$_{12}$ status and strengthen the case for routine B$_{12}$ tests

to be carried out as part of the full blood count. There is, however, another serious problem – the current serum B_{12} test is flawed for a number of reasons.

Problem 4: The limitations of the serum B_{12} test

Before we take a look at the failings of the current test to determine the B_{12} status in patients, we need to look at the evolution of the assays used before the introduction of the current test.

The first test that was used to assess the cobalamin (B_{12}) levels in patients used microbiology as its base:

> Historically, the first widely used clinical assay for cobala-min was a microbiologic assay. This assay utilized strains of *Lactobacillus leichmannii* or *Euglena gracilis* that depended on exogenously added cobalamin for growth.[vi] Cobalamin from a patient serum sample was extracted and incubated with the bacterium and growth was proportional to the amount of cobalamin present.[8]

The test was difficult to standardise across laboratories, and in the late 1970s a new test was developed and introduced that was based on radio-dilution. It immediately became clear that this new test was also not without problems:

> Subsequently, a radio-dilution assay was developed and widely adopted in the 1970s. Here, cobalamin was extracted from patient serum, converted to cyanocobalamin, and then mixed with radiolabeled 57cyanocobalamin. The level of radiolabeled cyanocobalamin binding to purified IF [intrin-sic factor – see page 25] was measured, and from this, the

---

[vi] One of the drawbacks of using microbiological assays was that antibiotics interfered with the bacterial growth and led to erroneous results.

amount of patient cyanocobalamin was calculated. This test also suffered several limitations, not the least of which was the use of radiolabeled isotopes in the clinical laboratory. In addition, it had been noted by the late 1970s that this assay may give falsely normal values of serum cobalamin levels in patients with pernicious anemia.[7]

One set of authors were not as polite:

Recent studies have demonstrated problems with the radiodilution assay method for measuring serum cobalamin (vitamin B_{12}) levels. We have found the standard commercial radiodilution kit assay to be totally ineffective in screening for cobalamin deficiency.[8]

Oh dear – it leads to the question why or how did it ever get adopted as a frontline test in the first place? Still, things improved with the introduction in the 1990s of the competitive-binding luminescence assay or CBLA – or did they? The CBLA is the assay which is widely used today to determine the B_{12} status in patients; and guess what – it's seriously flawed, giving up to 35% false high readings. This means that doctors who have requested a serum B_{12} test will end up believing that the patient's B_{12} status is fine or normal when in fact it is low or very low. As mentioned in the Introduction, the problem lies with the machines currently used to assess the blood sent for analysis.

And it's worse for patients who have true auto-immune pernicious anaemia because the patient's intrinsic factor antibodies interfere with the analysis taking place in the machine:

Today, vitamin B_{12} assays are primarily performed on automated analyzers that apply a method based on the competitive binding of serum vitamin B_{12} with reagent intrinsic factor. Many of these platforms have also been found to be inaccurate when serum containing intrinsic factor-blocking antibodies is analyzed. Disconcertingly, pernicious anemia is the most common cause of vitamin B_{12} deficiency, and up to 70% of patients with pernicious anemia have intrinsic factor-blocking antibodies.[9]

That quotation is from one of the two papers that I mentioned in the Introduction to this book that were published in the middle of 2012; both demonstrated that the current test to determine B_{12} status in patients was reporting false high levels of serum B_{12} in 22–35% of patients whose B_{12} status was assessed. With a quarter to a third of patients being told that their B_{12} status is fine, when it isn't, it's hardly surprising that so many patients are routinely being misdiagnosed or not diagnosed. This failure of the current test is not fair on patients, but equally not fair on physicians, because at the very least it is leading to unacceptable levels of wrong diagnosis that, in the worst cases, lead to severe and permanent nerve damage. I'll repeat what Ralph Carmel, the author of one of the papers, had to say about the current test:

Manufacturers, who have access to proprietary information, must instead transparently identify and permanently correct the defect or defects.[10]

New BCSH guidelines

I am pleased to say it's not all gloom and doom. There is now widespread acknowledgement that the current assay used to determine the B_{12} status of patients is flawed. See on the next page what the new BCSH guidelines on cobalamin and folate say about the test.

Summary of key recommendations[3]

• The clinical picture is the most important factor in assessing the significance of test results assessing cobalamin status since there is no 'gold standard' test to define deficiency.

• Serum cobalamin remains the first-line test currently, with additional second-line plasma methylmalonic acid to help clarify uncertainties of underlying biochemical/functional deficiencies. Serum holotranscobalamin has the potential as a first-line test, but an indeterminate 'grey area' may still exist. Plasma homocysteine may be helpful as a second-line test, but is less specific than methylmalonic acid. The availability of these second-line tests is currently limited.

• Definitive cut-off points to define clinical and subclinical deficiency states are not possible, given the variety of methodologies used and technical issues, and local reference ranges should be established.

• In the presence of discordance between the test result and strong clinical features of deficiency, treatment should not be delayed to avoid neurological impairment.

This is pretty strong language that is, in effect, telling doctors to ignore the results of the test if the patient has any of the symptoms of B$_{12}$ deficiency but the serum results do not support that. Now, I would like to be able to report that these guidelines have brought an end to the strict interpretation of test results that leads to so many members of the Pernicious Anaemia Society not receiving treatment, but it hasn't. Still we get telephone calls every day from patients who have a wide range of symptoms but whose test results show no deficiency. I really did believe that once the new guidelines were published it would bring about a sea-change in how patients were being treated – but with hindsight this was remarkably naïve of me. It will likely take many years before primary care physicians are fully conversant with the new guidelines. The Pernicious Anaemia Society is doing what it can to raise awareness among physicians using promotional materials, including posters and pop-up banners at events attended by doctors.

The new guidelines have been branded as something of a paper tiger by some – but I don't think they are. For the first time there is recognition that there is something seriously amiss with the way in which B_{12} status is assessed. For those who have classic megaloblastic anaemia it is usually quite a straightforward procedure to make a firm diagnosis, but, as the new guidelines acknowledge:

> However, the majority of patients do not have such a clear cut picture. Neurological presentation (peripheral neuropathy, sub-acute combined degeneration of the cord) may occur in the absence of haematological changes, and early treatment is essential to avoid permanent neurological disability. Low cobalamin levels of uncertain significance may occur with non-specific symptoms and no anaemia. Furthermore, patients with strong clinical features of cobalamin deficiency may have serum cobalamin levels which lie within the reference range (false normal cobalamin level).[3]

New B_{12} tests

So, it is now generally agreed that there are serious problems with the way in which the B_{12} status of patients is assessed, but what can be done about this problem? Well, the BCSH's guidelines don't offer any definitive solution but do mention other tests that could be used instead of the current serum B_{12} test, or in conjunction with the current test. These include methyl malonic acid (MMA), total homocysteine (tHcy) and holotranscobalamin (HoloTC).[vii] Unfortunately, only one of these is a serious contender to become the standard test. In the box is what the BCSH says about them.

BCSH guidance on alternative tests

• **MMA** – The plasma MMA is raised in cobalamin deficiency. However, plasma MMA may be falsely elevated in subjects with renal disease, small bowel bacterial overgrowth and haemoconcentration. Despite these limitations, exceptionally high levels of plasma MMA (>0.75 μmol/l) almost invariably indicate cobalamin deficiency.

• **tHcy** – However, tHcy is not specific to cobalamin deficiency as concentrations of tHcy are also elevated in folate deficiency, B$_6$ deficiency and in patients with renal failure, hypothyroidism and as a result of certain genetic polymorphisms.

• **HoloTC** – Holotranscobalamin (HoloTC), the 'active' fraction of plasma cobalamin, may be more specific than serum cobalamin levels, and an immunoassay for this fraction is now available. In clinical research studies, the HoloTC assay performs better than serum cobalamin assay in assessing deficiency based on MMA levels and red cell cobalamin levels as reference assays.

The HoloTC test

Holotranscobalamin measures the 'active' form of B$_{12}$. Serum B$_{12}$ – the amount of B$_{12}$ in the blood serum – measures the total

---

[vii] The use of bone marrow examination was ruled out.

amount of B_{12} but there are two distinct forms of the vitamin. Holohaptocorrin is the 'inactive' form that doesn't play any part in the biological process that takes place in making healthy red blood cells, while its cousin, holotranscobalamin, does. What this new test therefore does is differentiate between the 'active' B_{12} and the 'inactive' B_{12}. Surprisingly, or perhaps not so surprisingly, up to 90% of total B_{12} can be of the inactive sort. On the face of it, this newcomer seems to be the answer to the problem of assessing patients' B_{12} status accurately; yet even this test has its critics and it will have to prove itself by undergoing a series of trials and assessments before it is fully accepted and becomes the 'mainstream' test for B_{12}. The new BCSH guidelines are, however, generally optimistic:

> Since samples for HoloTC analysis do not need any special pre-analytical preparation, and can be stored for batch analysis, it appears to be a strong candidate for future routine first line assessment of cobalamin deficiency, particularly if costs of the test become favourable.

Somebody who knows about the 'Active B_{12} Test' is Dr Dominic Harrington who is a Consultant Clinical Scientist based at St Thomas' Hospital in London, where the new B_{12} test has been available since 2011. He is also Reader in Diagnostic Haematology at King's College London, and Scientific Director for Viapath. I asked him what he thought of the current B_{12} test. He explained:

> Most commonly, vitamin B_{12} status is evaluated through the measurement of vitamin B_{12} in serum by automated platforms based on competitive-binding luminescence technologies. Status is estimated from the abundance of vitamin B_{12} in the circulation. It is important to be mindful that the current test measures vitamin B_{12} that is bound to two different binding proteins, transcobalamin II and haptocorrin. Therefore the result generated by the laboratory reflects 'total' vitamin B_{12}.

What this means is that B$_{12}$ binds to two types of protein and the current test doesn't differentiate between these two forms of B$_{12}$ in the blood. Dr Harrington went on:

> We need to remember that the current test gives no indication of vitamin B$_{12}$ utilisation by target tissues – just its abundance in the blood. It is widely accepted that a high rate of false negative results are generated by this test. [Put simply – this means the current test is not accurate but there's more] Some patient groups are affected more than others. One important example includes false normal vitamin B$_{12}$ results that are reported in patients with high titre intrinsic factor antibodies.

What he means by that is that, as I mentioned above, if a person has lots of intrinsic factor antibodies – that is, they have pernicious anaemia – there is a good chance that their serum B$_{12}$ will appear to be normal. And if you thought things couldn't get worse, they do:

> Another factor to consider is the variation in the performance of the commonly available assays. Patient results are partly dependent on which analytical platform is being used by the local laboratory.

This means, in other words, that not only is the current test flawed, but the different machines produced by different manufacturers do not all perform to the same standards. There are obviously some serious issues that need addressing here. So what about this new Active B$_{12}$ test? I asked Dr Harrington what would be the advantage of replacing the current test with the new one:

> The new 'Active B$_{12}$' test only measures the abundance of the physiologically active form of cobalamin (i.e. vitamin B$_{12}$ bound to transcobalamin) and ignores the fraction bound to haptocorrin. Use of the 'Active B$_{12}$' assay is increas-

ingly widespread in Australia, Austria, Canada, Germany, Holland, Nordic countries, the UK and Switzerland.

So, the Active B_{12} is the form of B_{12} that plays an active biological role in the body?

> Although in blood around 80% of vitamin B_{12} is carried by haptocorrin, extra-hepatic cellular receptors for this form have not been identified. We know that circulatory levels of haptocorrin decline slowly in response to negative vitamin B_{12} balance, i.e. when metabolic requirements exceed absorption of dietary vitamin B_{12}. It is actually vitamin B_{12} bound to transcobalamin that is metabolically active (commercially coined 'Active B_{12}'). Transcobalamin transports about 4 nmol/l of vitamin B_{12} into cells each day whereas haptocorrin transports just 0.1 nmol/l.

It must make sense then to measure only the active B_{12} as the other form is not very good at doing what it should be doing. However, what if the person being tested has high levels of intrinsic factor antibodies? Would their active B_{12} appear normal even if that wasn't the case? Dr Harrington replied:

> A decrease in 'Active B_{12}' levels is thought to be the earliest indicator of negative vitamin B_{12} balance. The new assay does not appear to generate false normal vitamin B_{12} levels in subjects with high titre[viii] intrinsic factor antibody.

Early indications are that this new test will identify a lot more patients as having a B_{12} deficiency than are currently being recognised, and that can only be a good thing. However, there are those who are sceptical about the new test offering the solution to an increasingly recognised problem with the current test. They think that:

[viii] 'Titre' relates to a concentration of a solution.

It is highly controversial and premature, because too little is known about what factors influence holotranscobalamin levels. Detailed, clinically relevant studies are scarce, and those which do exist are often less positive in their recommendations on its use than the clinically uninformative biochemical surveys of subclinical deficiency, which show marginal advantages for the use of holotranscobalamin.[11]

Problem 5: Understanding subclinical B$_{12}$ deficiency

A caregiver must manage a sub-clinically deficient patient with pernicious anemia as a cause quite differently and pay closer attention than to a similar patient without it.[12]

Lately there has been an acceptance that there is a 'grey area' where patients experience the symptoms of B$_{12}$ deficiency but have serum B$_{12}$ levels above the level used to diagnose a deficiency. It's a murky area and so it would be a good idea to begin with a definition of what subclinical means. The *Oxford Concise Medical Dictionary* defines subclinical as 'describing a disease that is suspected but is not sufficiently developed to produce definite signs and symptoms in the patient'. In this context, the patient would be experiencing a few or many of the symptoms of B$_{12}$ deficiency but their serum B$_{12}$ levels would be above what is normally regarded as the threshold used to mark a deficiency. In these situations, some doctors will realise that an injection of B$_{12}$ is cheap, safe and readily available and it might be worthwhile to commence replacement therapy and see if the patient's symptoms go away or at least become less severe. This is often referred to as a 'therapeutic trial' and I truly wish more doctors would follow this route as it would mean that around half of the telephone calls that I take on a daily basis would end.

Instead, what usually happens is that the doctor refuses to provide the patient with any treatment, usually asking the patient to 'come back in six months and we'll check your levels again', presumably in the hope that the patient's serum B_{12} will have dropped below the threshold used to show a deficiency and the patient can then proceed to receive treatment. Patients, however, are not stupid and will usually start treating themselves, either using injections or the increasingly popular sub-lingual sprays or lozenges. And this means that their serum B_{12} levels will increase dramatically, meaning they'll never receive any prescribed treatment from their doctor.

So, what measurement of B_{12} in blood serum constitutes a deficiency? Well, a good place to look would be the new guidelines from the BCSH , but unfortunately this doesn't get us very far. They are not helpful here:

> It is not entirely clear what should be regarded as a clinically normal serum cobalamin level, although it has been proposed that a serum cobalamin of less than 200 ng/l (148 pmol/l)[ix] would have a sensitivity of diagnosing 97% of true cobalamin deficiency.[13]

Now take a look at that sentence again. It states that 'it has been proposed' – not defined or agreed what would constitute a cobalamin deficiency – but 'proposed'. No wonder that 'it is not entirely clear' what constitutes a normal cobalamin level. So, who should make the final decision as to what figure marks a deficiency? The BCSH says:

> Establishment of reference ranges by individual laboratories can be challenging since the serum cobalamin level can be affected by many variables i.e. diet, pregnancy, vitamin supplements, contraceptive pill, metformin etc.

[ix] The figures given represent nanograms per millilitre – there are 1 billion nanograms in a gram – it's a measurement of weight. Pmol refers to picomoles which measure how much of a chemical substance is present in a litre of blood serum – in this case cobalamin. 1 pmol/l = 1.355 ng/l.

Who should take responsibility for establishing these reference ranges? The BCSH point the finger at the manufacturers:

> They [the reference ranges] are best conducted by robust studies, accounting for such variables, by the manufacturer.

And the committee goes on to say:

> The laboratories may then report their results adjusted in relation to assay bias of the consensus mean in UKNEQAS[x] surveys.

Note the use of the word 'may' – not 'should' or 'ought' but 'may'.

I may be being a little unfair on the new guidelines. They do, after all, acknowledge that there is a problem with the way in which cobalamin deficiency is currently investigated and they do, in their recommendations, state that all future laboratory tests for cobalamin should in future always be given in pmol/l which should bring an end to any confusion in interpreting the results. And they also mark a line in the sand when it comes to establishing a lower threshold that could define a deficiency:

> A serum cobalamin cut-off level of either 148 pmol/l (200 ng/l) or one derived from a local reference range should be used as evidence of cobalamin deficiency in the presence of a strong clinical suspicion.

Note that they leave room for individual laboratories to set their own figure – 'or one derived from a local reference range'.

It is good that the BCSH has identified that things are not all black and white when it comes to identifying a B_{12} deficiency, and I

---

[x] The United Kingdom National External Quality Assessment Service for Microbiology.

believe that, whilst the new guidelines are not perfect, they do go a long way to raising awareness among medical professionals of the limitations of the current test. They do also make recommendations for the introduction of what could be more promising assays. Just how long it will take for these recommendations to be introduced is impossible to say. In the meantime, I and my volunteers will be left with the thankless daily task of trying to explain to patients why their doctor refuses to offer them treatment because their B_{12} results are just one or two digits above the threshold used to determine a deficiency even though they have a whole raft of symptoms.

And all of this is further complicated by the fact that some commentators believe the current threshold to determine any deficiency is far too low anyway and should be raised. This is a view that is often put forward by patients whose serum B_{12} measurement is above, often well above, the parameter used to define a diagnosis of any deficiency. Raising the current threshold might be a positive way forward and would probably help identify early those patients who are deficient in the vitamin:

> We believe that the traditional cut-off value of 148 pmol/l
> is too low. We suggest that physicians should consider
> treating patients who show symptoms but have vitamin B_{12}
> levels above this value, particularly those in the low-normal
> range up to approximately 300 pmol/l, to see whether their
> symptoms are relieved.[3]

If this was to happen and the numerical value used to identify any B_{12} deficiency was double what it is today, there would be a number of consequences. Firstly, and most importantly as far as I am concerned, it would mean that a far greater number of people would be investigated to find out if their deficiency was caused by pernicious anaemia. Secondly, and linked to the first consequence, there should be a significant decrease in the time it takes for patients with pernicious anaemia to obtain a correct diagnosis. Remember that

14% of patients responding to the survey waited over 10 years for a diagnosis. A third consequence follows on from the second – it would improve the quality of life for hundreds of thousands, maybe millions, of people who are currently in this 'subclinical' no-man's land who are experiencing many of the symptoms of a deficiency in B$_{12}$ but whose serum levels of the vitamin remain stubbornly, marginally above what is now the threshold value used to determine a deficiency. It may be a blunt instrument, but doubling the current threshold value would mean bringing an end to the current problems in receiving a diagnosis of being deficient in B$_{12}$, even if it would mean an even bigger membership base for the Pernicious Anaemia Society.

Problem 6: Understanding the effect of B$_{12}$ analogues

It's often said that if you gave a certain problem to five economists you would get five different solutions. It's a bit like that with the strange world of analogues – ask scientists to define what an analogue is and you get a variety of different replies; some even let out a gentle whistle and shake their head from side to side much as a car mechanic does just before he gives you an estimate for the cost of repairing your car. That said, we can define an analogue as follows: 'In chemistry, a structural analogue, also known as a chemical analogue or simply analogue, is a compound having a structure similar to that of another one, but differing from it in respect of a certain component.'[14]

Analogues occur throughout biology – they are slight variations on 'the real thing'. So an analogue of vitamin B$_{12}$ will be similar to a molecule of real B$_{12}$ but will be subtly different. And this a problem, because analogues of B$_{12}$ will be included in any test result to determine B$_{12}$ status in patients but they won't be 'real' B$_{12}$. Does this matter? It's difficult to say but it was certainly a problem in the past when the microbiological assay was used:

> The recent introduction of radioassays for 'true' cobalamin, as opposed to cobalamin and its analogues, has resulted in significantly lower levels of cobalamin being found in patients with folate deficiency.[15]

The extent to which the CBLA measures analogues as well as true cobalamins is something that I haven't been able to find out. That said, it seems likely or even certain that some analogues of B_{12} will be included in any evaluation of B_{12} in patients' blood, though whether this is a significant problem is not known.

Summary

In summary then, it can be said that the current way in which patients' B_{12} is evaluated is seriously flawed or, as one commentator puts it: 'Functional cobalamin deficiency can thus occur at any serum level.'[16] Thankfully there is now widespread acknowledgment of the failings of the CBLA and in Chapter 8, which is a much more cheerful and optimistic chapter than this one, we shall examine the latest developments in this area.

Now, let's assume that a patient has acknowledged his or her symptoms and has talked to his or her GP who has immediately suspected B_{12} deficiency and questioned the patient about his or her diet and ruled that out as being a possible cause of the condition. The doctor has then checked the patient's file to see if any gastric surgery has taken place in the past and found that no procedures have been performed. However, when the patient has been questioned about his or her family history of pernicious anaemia, the GP has been told that two family members have been diagnosed with pernicious anaemia in the past. At that moment, a light goes on in the physician's head and he or she immediately orders a full blood count and folate and B_{12} test. The B_{12} test comes back as low and so the doctor is then faced with the possibility that the patient's low B_{12} is caused by pernicious anaemia; he/she orders the anti-intrinsic factor antibody test to confirm a diagnosis of pernicious anaemia. If the test comes back as 'negative' for the antibody, this means the patient doesn't have pernicious anaemia – or does it? You see, the intrinsic factor antibody test is also seriously flawed; and it is to this issue that we will now turn in the next chapter.

References

1 Beck WS. Neuropsychiatric consequences of cobalamin deficiency. *Advanced Institute of Medicine* 1991; 36:33–56.

2 Lindenbaum J, Healton EB, et al. Neuropsychiatric disorders caused by cobalamin deficiency in the absence of anemia or macrocytosis. *New England Journal of Medicine* 1988; 318(26):1720–1728.

3 Devalia, V, Hamilton M, Molloy A. Guidelines for the diagnosis and treatment of cobalamin and folate disorders. *British Journal of Haematology* 2014; 166(4):497.

4 Carmel R. Current concepts in cobalamin deficiency. *Annual Review of Medicine* 2000; 51:357–375.

5 Scarpa E, Candiotto L, Sartori R, Radossi P, Maschio N, Tagariello G. Undetected vitamin B_{12} deficiency due to false normal assay results. *Blood Transfusion* 2013; 11(4):627–629. doi: 10.2450/2012.0183-12

6 De Walsn P, Tairou F, Van Allen M, Uh S-H, Lowry B, Sibbald B, Evans J A, Van den Hof M C, Zimmer P, Crowley M, Fernandez B, Lee N S, Niyonsenga T. Reduction in neural-tube defects after folic acid fortification in Canada. *New England Journal of Medicine* 2007; 357:135-142.

7 National Diet and Nutrition Survey: Blood folate results for the UK, Scotland, Northern Ireland (Years 1 to 4 combined) and Wales (Years 2 to 5 combined). Published by Public Health England. https://www.gov.uk/government/uploads/system/uploads/attach-

ment_data/file/414745/NDNS_Y1_4_Folate_report.pdf (Accessed 19 July 2015.

8 Oberley MJ, Yang DT. Laboratory testing for cobalamin deficiency in megaloblastic anemia. *American Journal of Hematology* 2013; 88:522–526.

9 Ibid.

10 Carmel R, Agrawal YP. Failures of cobalamin assays in pernicious anaemia. *New England Journal of Medicine* 2012; 367(4):385–386.

11 Cohen JKL, Donaldson RM Jr. Unreliability of radiodilution assays as screening tests for cobalamin (vitamin B_{12}) deficiency. *Journal of American Medical Association* 1980; 244(17):1942–1945.

12 Yang D, Cook R. Spurious elevations of vitamin B_{12} with pernicious anemia. *New England Journal of Medicine* 2012; 366:1742–1743.

13 Ibid ref 3.

14 Carmel R, Agrawal Y. (Authors' Reply) More on failures of cobalamin assays in pernicious anemia. *New England Journal of Medicine* 2012; 367(16):1569-1571.

15 Carmel R, Sarrai M. Diagnosis and management of clinical and subclinical cobalamin deficiency: advances and controversies. *Current Hematology Reports* 2006; 5(1):23-33.

16 Ibid ref 3.

17 Smith D, Refsum H. Do we need to reconsider the desirable blood level of vitamin B_{12}? *Journal of Internal Medicine* 2011; 271(2):179–182.doi: 10.1111/j.1365–2796.2011.02485.

18 Willett P, Barnard JM, Downs GM. Chemical similarity searching. *Journal of Chemical Information and Computer Science* 1998; 38:983–996. doi:10.1021/ci9800211.

19 Johnson AM, Maggiora GM. *Concepts and Applications of Molecular Similarity.* New York: John Wiley & Sons; 1990.

20 Nikolova N, Jaworska J. Approaches to measure chemical similarity – a review. *QSAR & Combinatorial Science* 2003; 22(9-10):1006–1026.doi:10.1002/qsar.200330831.

21 Sheppard K, Ryrie D. Changes in serum levels of cobalamin and cobalamin analogues in folate deficiency. *Scandinavian Journal of Haematology* 1980; 25(5):401–406.

22 Andre ES, Serraj K, Zhu J, Vermorken AJM. The pathophysiology of elevated vitamin B$_{12}$ in clinical practice. *Quarterly Journal of Medicine* 2013; 106(6):505.

Chapter 4

Problems in diagnosing pernicious anaemia

Early attempts to understand pernicious anaemia

One November morning in 1927 at a hospital in Boston USA, Dr William Bosworth Castle was preparing to regurgitate 300 grams of raw hamburger patties that he had eaten an hour earlier. He stuck his fingers down his throat and successfully brought up the semi-digested meat. He then began to adjust the semi-liquid to a pH of 2.5–3.5 using hydrochloric acid and set it aside to incubate for six hours before passing the liquid through a fine muslin cloth. He then set off on his rounds armed with the rank-smelling liquid in one hand, and a pile of consent forms in the other.

The previous year George Minot working at Harvard University had fed raw or lightly cooked liver to his patients who were dying from pernicious anaemia. Nobody knew quite why the raw liver allowed the patients to live, but for the first time the pernicious part of the title of the disease had become somewhat redundant. As we now know, the raw liver contained very high levels of vitamin B_{12}, and some of the B_{12}, because there was so much of it, found its way into the bloodstream 'passively'.

Dr Castle wanted to know why normal healthy patients didn't have to eat raw liver. It was his supposition that something in the gastric juices in the stomach allowed such people to absorb something from food that made this possible. It turned out he was correct. The patients on his wards suffering from pernicious anaemia were, presumably, most grateful for the raw liver that they were being fed daily given that the outcome offered by the alternative was so final. They must have taken quite some persuading to agree to test Dr Castle's new treatment, especially as this involved having a rubber tube inserted into their stomach via their mouth.

Dr Castle didn't tell his patients what he was giving them – any questions relating to what exactly was going to be fed into the tube were answered in vague euphemisms whilst gesticulating wildly to his wide-eyed patients clutching their consent forms.[1] Obviously, however well-intentioned Castle's study was, it is hard to imagine any such covert experiment being permitted today, or at least I like to think so. Was Dr Castle aware that perhaps he was pushing the boundaries of acceptability in scientific enquiry by not fully informing his patients? The answer is probably illustrated by the following:

> When he submitted his initial studies of intrinsic factor to the Warren Triennial Prize Committee at the MGH in 1928, Castle was bound by rules requiring anonymity. He identified his winning entry with the regal disclaimer, 'Honi soit qui mal y pense'.

'Honi soit qui mal y pense' is the motto of the UK's Order of the Garter and literally translated means 'shame on him who thinks evil of it'.

The important point is that Castle realised there was something in human gastric juices that needed to be present to ensure that the patient derived benefit from animal products and, as I have said, he called this 'something' *intrinsic factor* – the food in question being the *extrinsic factor*. It was to be another 20 years before vitamin B$_{12}$ was isolated, but from the late 1920s on the secrets of B_{12} began to be unearthed. However, it is worth noting that it wasn't until the early 1970s that the complete picture of intrinsic factor became known.

Not long after Castle's famous regurgitation project he, along with other doctors produced:

> a 'domestic liver extract' that could be injected safely either intramuscularly or (given slowly) intravenously. This discovery was not only of great practical merit but also led to the provocative finding that the protein-free, water-soluble principle was far more potent, unit for unit, when given parenterally [that is, directly into the blood stream] than when taken orally.[2]

We'll look at the issues surrounding the treatment of pernicious anaemia in Chapter 5, but for now we will concentrate on the problems of testing for pernicious anaemia.

Testing for intrinsic factor

To determine whether a patient's low B_{12} was or is caused by pernicious anaemia, doctors must find out whether the patient has intrinsic factor in his or her stomach. To do this, modern tests don't look for intrinsic factor directly, but instead search for an antibody that neutralises the intrinsic factor – the anti-intrinsic factor antibody test (usually abbreviated to intrinsic factor antibody or IFA). Why is this? Why don't doctors investigate whether the patient has intrinsic factor in his or her stomach but instead look for an antibody to the protein? It was a question that I put to someone who has devoted a large part of his life to investigating pernicious anaemia, the renowned haematologist Dr Ralph Carmel from New York. He replied as follows:

> The question about IF assay is logical because IF testing,

although not perfect, is almost certainly the most reliable test of all for PA. The test has fallen by the wayside because it is semi-invasive, uncomfortable, and labor-intensive. A nasogastric tube[i] must be inserted into the stomach after the patient has fasted overnight, it must be properly positioned, it must lie in place and be continuously aspirated for some time, often an hour, because 'spot' samples are often misleading; reliable collection requires stimulation of the stomach by hormone injection (IF can sometimes be absent in the resting stomach but become abundant after the stomach has been stimulated) and the ideal hormone/agent can have side effects. Furthermore, the collected gastric juice must be neutralized with careful pH manipulation to prevent degradation of IF in vitro. Moreover, almost no labs are capable of measuring IF accurately today.

And that is why doctors don't try to see whether patients have or have not got any intrinsic factor but rely on two other tests – the intrinsic factor antibody test and/or the gastric parietal cell antibody test. To understand what these are we need to go back to the stomach and in particular to the lining of the stomach wall.

How the stomach works

As we learnt in Chapter 1, the stomach is only one of the digestive organs that play a part in the digestive process. It is also not the first stage – that occurs when you masticate (chew) food and mix it with saliva. Food that's been chewed and mixed with saliva is known as 'bolus'. Bolus travels down the oesophagus and enters into the stomach via a sphincter muscle (the lower oesophageal sphincter) which only allows food to travel one way (downwards), unless, of course, you want to regurgitate raw hamburger meat (see Figure 4.1).

[i] A tube inserted into the stomach via the nose.

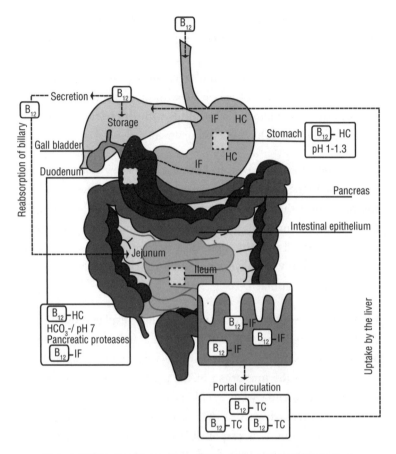

Figure 4.1 The digestive system showing the uptake of vitamin B$_{12}$.
(IF = intrinsic factor; HC = haptocorrin; TC = transcobalamin.)

The stomach contains a network of blood vessels and nerves (plexuses) that control the secretions of the stomach lining and the motion of the stomach muscles. The secretions include protein-digesting enzymes (proteases, including pepsin), hydrochloric acid and intrinsic factor. It is the hydrochloric acid that is actually responsible for releasing bound B$_{12}$ from the food. Intrinsic factor is produced in a part of the stomach called the 'fundus'. The fundus is lined with 'parietal cells' and it is these that produce the intrinsic factor. This combination of chemicals is known as the *gastric juices*; these are churned into bolus by muscular contractions of the stomach wall and the result is a watery mixture called 'chyme'. It's a complicated procedure with some very complex chemistry involved which we don't need to go into, but we do need to be aware that it is in the stomach that the intrinsic factor binds with B_{12} released from any animal products that have been consumed.

It takes anywhere between 40 minutes and a few hours for food processing in the stomach to be completed. The B_{12}/intrinsic factor combination is then part of the chyme that makes its way into the first part of the small intestine – the duodenum. It is in the various parts of the small intestine that most nutrients are absorbed; only water (if the body is dehydrated), and aspirin, as it happens, are absorbed in the stomach.[ii]

What I have described here is a very simplistic explanation of a fascinating and highly complicated process that involves all manner of biological and chemical actions – and, as we learnt in Chapter 1, the stomach is only the first organ in the process of digestion. Again, we don't need to know what exactly takes place in these organs, but suffice it to say, each part of the small intestine – the duodenum, jejunum and ileum – is responsible for absorbing all manner of nutrients and minerals from food. What is of particular interest to us in this chapter is the ileum, which is the final part of the small intestine, as it is in the ileum that the B_{12}/intrinsic factor combination is absorbed into the bloodstream.

Just how the B_{12} gets into the bloodstream is again a highly complex procedure, but put simply the IF/B_{12} complex is recognised by

[ii] Gastric acid is needed to release B_{12} from food, which is why patients taking antacid medications, including proton pump inhibitors, run the risk of becoming B_{12} deficient. The terms 'achlorhydria' and 'hypochlorhydria' refer to lack of gastric acid.

ileal receptors on cells in the wall of the ileum and is passed into the bloodstream where the vitamin then binds with a 'transporter' called transcobalamin II (TcII/B_{12}) and sets off to help build healthy red blood cells.

Testing for parietal cell antibodies

Now we need to rewind a little further. It is in the stomach that the intrinsic factor is produced by the parietal cells and intrinsic fator is needed for B_{12} absorption. Consequently, if those parietal cells are not doing what they are supposed to do then there will be no intrinsic factor to bind to the B_{12} that has been released from food by the stomach acid. You were first introduced to gastric atrophy (or atrophic gastritis – they mean the same thing) in Chapter 2 and learnt that this is a disease that affects the lining of the stomach causing it to become inflamed. There are two causes of atrophic gastritis:

- One is *Helicobacter pylori* infection. *H. pylori* is a bacterium that can avoid being dissolved by the stomach's hydrochloric acid by burrowing into the gastric wall. It is incredibly common, with around 50% of the world's population having it, though up to 80% of those infected will have none of the symptoms associated with the microbe (stomach pains, nausea, bloating, belching, and sometimes vomiting or black stools).
- The second, and one that is perhaps of more interest to us, is autoimmune atrophic gastritis, where the body produces antibodies that attack the parietal cells – parietal cell antibodies.

So, gastric atrophy will interfere with the production of intrinsic factor, without which we cannot absorb any B_{12} that has been released from food into the bloodstream. Logically then, testing for parietal cell antibodies would be an excellent tool to investigate whether a patient has pernicious anaemia. There are some doctors who believe this is so:

Testing for gastric parietal cell antibodies is an appropriate screening test for pernicious anaemia, with intrinsic factor antibodies reserved for confirmatory testing, or in patients with other autoantibodies that mask the GPC pattern; B12 levels are not related to autoantibody status.[3]

However, new guidelines issued by the British Committee for Standards in Haematology (BCSH) (see page xvi) aren't as enthusiastic:

Gastric parietal cell antibodies (GPC antibodies) have a low specificity for the presence of pernicious anaemia since, despite being positive in 80% of pernicious anaemia subjects, they are also positive in 10% of normal individuals. Positive gastric parietal cell antibodies may cause gastric acid achlorhydria[iii] and progression to pernicious anaemia may occur. However, a positive GPC antibody test is not definitive for pernicious anaemia.[4]

The recommendations section of these guidelines is more to the point:

Anti-gastric parietal cell antibody testing for diagnosing pernicious anaemia is not recommended.

This rejection of parietal cell antibodies as being a test for pernicious anaemia has been widely debated on various social media sites because a substantial number of patients have been diagnosed as having pernicious anaemia because they tested positive for gastric parietal cell antibodies, and so for them the test is a valid one. However, as far as the BCSH is concerned it is not 'specific' enough. I am not a doctor and consequently don't feel it appropriate for me to comment; after all, the members of the committee making the recommendations are highly skilled, experienced and esteemed professionals and I'm sure there was considerable deliberation and discussion before they made that recommendation.

So, the test to detect intrinsic factor is not viable and the test for antibodies to the parietal cells is not recommended, which leaves just one other test that can be used to determine whether the patient is producing intrinsic factor but is also producing an antibody that 'kills off' any intrinsic factor that he or she has produced – the anti-intrinsic factor antibody test.

Anti-intrinsic factor antibody test

This test makes one very large assumption – that the patient's parietal cells are working fine and he or she *is* producing intrinsic factor. The test therefore seeks to identify antibodies in the patient's blood that would explain why he/she is lacking vitamin B_{12}. Of course, if the patient doesn't have any gastric atrophy there is no reason to suppose he or she wouldn't be producing intrinsic factor and so antibodies to the IF would be a logical explanation for the lack of B_{12} and would lead to the physician diagnosing a case of pernicious anaemia. Unfortunately, there is a problem – the test is not in any way accurate, and I know from personal experience that this is the case; I tested negative for the antibodies twice before eventually testing strongly positive. And I'm not the only one who knows this – the BCSH also know; here's what they have to say about it:

> The finding of a low total serum cobalamin level may be further evaluated by testing for anti-intrinsic factor antibody (IFAB). If positive, the test has a high positive predictive value (95%) for the presence of pernicious anaemia.

So far so good – it means that if the patient's blood shows that he or she has intrinsic factor antibodies then it's 95% certain that pernicious anaemia is the cause of the patient's symptoms. There is, however, a problem – and it's a big one. Often the test will return a negative result even though the patient does have the antibodies:

IFAB is positive in 40–60% of cases i.e. low sensitivity, and the finding of a negative intrinsic factor antibody assay does not therefore rule out pernicious anaemia (hereafter referred to as AbNegPA).

So, around half the people tested will be told that they don't have any antibody when in fact they may well have it. And there's more:

In addition, the positivity rate increases with age and in certain racial groups [Latino-Americans and African-Americans].

What this means is that testing negative for intrinsic factor antibody does not mean that you *don't* have pernicious anaemia. And that means that a great many people who are told they don't have the condition in reality do, and that, unfortunately the only test that is available to give a definitive diagnosis of pernicious anaemia is not really fit for purpose. As one haematologist told me, the test 'nearly always comes back as negative'. This is a major problem because patients who have low serum B$_{12}$ should be further tested to discover whether that deficiency is caused by lack of intrinsic factor. If the test comes back as being negative for intrinsic factor antibodies, then the patient doesn't receive a firm diagnosis and is in a sort of no-man's-land, or, perhaps more accurately, in purgatory. The office of the Pernicious Anaemia Society receives calls from patients on a daily basis who have been given no explanation for their B$_{12}$ deficiency.

The Schilling test

The failings in the diagnostic tests for vitamin B$_{12}$ deficiency and its causes are adversely affecting the lives of thousands, maybe millions, of people throughout the world. Are there any solutions? Before these modern tests were developed there used to be a test that used radioactive B$_{12}$ to see if patients were able to absorb the vitamin in their gut.

The Schilling test was named after the American doctor who developed the process in the early 1950s – Dr Robert F Schilling. The test is no longer available in most laboratories because of the difficulty in sourcing radioactive B_{12}, which is no longer manufactured on any scale. The test involved two different stages to find the cause of any B_{12} deficiency.

- **Stage 1**: The patient received a dose of radioactive B_{12} by mouth and a non-radioactive injection. He/she then collected his or her urine over 24 hours which was sent to a laboratory where it was analysed to see if the patient had absorbed the oral B_{12}. If the test showed that less than 10% of the radioactive B_{12} had been absorbed, then further investigation was carried out to find out why the patient hadn't absorbed the oral B_{12}. The injection was given to 'saturate' the patient with B_{12} and so any oral B_{12} should have been absorbed in the gut and then passed out in the urine as being surplus to requirements, so to speak. If less than 10% was excreted in the urine, it meant that the patient simply hadn't absorb the B_{12} and it would instead be passed out in faeces. So, if there was less than 10% of the radioactive B_{12} in the urine, then stage 2 of the test began three to seven days later.
- **Stage 2**: The patient was given radioactive B_{12} and oral intrinsic factor. If the urine then showed an increase in the radioactive B_{12} this meant that the patient was now absorbing the B_{12} and must therefore be lacking his/her own intrinsic factor and therefore had pernicious anaemia. If the test still showed less than 10% of the radioactive B_{12} in the urine, the patient was investigated further for coeliac disease, biliary disease, Whipple's disease, small bowel bacterial overgrowth syndrome, fish tapeworm infestation, or liver disease.

The test wasn't perfect (imagine having exactly 10% of the radioactive B_{12} in your urine – what would happen then?) and it was time-consuming and costly. It can still be performed but special measures would have to be made for this to happen – you'd have to make some radioactive B$_{12}$ for a start. I know that one professor spent six months trying to source some but couldn't find any in existence. Anyway, the Schilling test was the test that was used to diagnose pernicious anaemia for 40 years but is now not available.

Using symptoms not tests to diagnose pernicious anaemia

So where does that leave us? The Schilling test is no longer available and the current CBLA is unreliable. Perhaps it is time for doctors to revert to diagnosing pernicious anaemia from the symptoms alone, as they had for many decades before assays were invented to confirm a diagnosis – but I'm aware that that's not going to happen. Modern medicine, like society in general, is being led by technological advances, especially in the relatively new field of nanoscience (more of this in Chapter 7) and so diagnosing on symptoms alone and relying on the individual physician's experience and knowledge would be seen to be a retrograde step. However, there are some doctors practising in the UK who have known for many years that the current tests are flawed and rely on their knowledge and experience to make a diagnosis based solely on the patient's symptoms.

It is all too easy to point an accusing finger at clinicians and accuse them of failing to listen to what a patient is telling them and instead paying too much attention to a computer-generated printout of the test results. However, modern technologies in laboratories are, for the most part, reliable and trustworthy and during the many years spent training for their vocation, junior doctors are instructed to make their diagnosis on clinical evidence; and that's what the test for intrinsic factor antibody is – clinical evidence. And whilst there is growing acknowledgement that the test is flawed, it is still not universally known that the current test to determine whether a patient has pernicious anaemia is unreliable. Again, the new BCSH guidelines address this problem by recommending:

> Patients negative for intrinsic factor antibody, with no other causes of deficiency, may still have pernicious anaemia and should be treated as anti-intrinsic factor antibody negative pernicious anaemia. Lifelong therapy should be continued in the presence of an objective clinical response.

Once again, it's not all doom and gloom. There are doctors who are aware of the limitations of the IFA test and who are prepared to diagnose patients as having pernicious anaemia even if the results of the assay do not show any intrinsic factor antibodies present in the patient's blood. I know of doctors who will make a diagnosis on symptoms alone because I regularly receive telephone calls or emails from patients whose test results do not support a diagnosis and who will have often spent many years trying to find an explanation for their symptoms. For some reason or another they happen upon a doctor who *will* diagnose them as having pernicious anaemia, and that diagnosis will be based not only on their symptoms but also on other factors, including one very strong indicator – a family history of pernicious anaemia.

Genetics and pernicious anaemia

One set of questions from the Pernicious Anaemia Society's survey addressed the issue of heredity and asked if the respondent had other family members who had received a firm diagnosis of pernicious anaemia. The results were as follows:

- parent (15%)
- grandparent (15%)
- sibling (6%)
- child (2%)

- uncle/aunt (9%)
- cousin (4%).

These figures need to be taken in the context that we know that it is often difficult to get a firm diagnosis of pernicious anaemia and some patients would have ticked more than one box. That said, it can be seen that pernicious anaemia can run in families. I spoke to an Australian member recently whose maternal grandmother had been diagnosed with pernicious anaemia, as had her mother, aunt, two sisters and a (young) cousin.

Dr Siddharth Banka is a Clinical Senior Lecturer at the Institute of Human Development, University of Manchester and a Consultant in genetic medicine. He has long been interested in how pernicious anaemia occurs within families and has used members of the Pernicious Anaemia Society as participants in a series of studies investigating the genetics of the disease. I asked him what he and his team had uncovered.

> Pernicious anaemia is thought to be a multi-factorial condition, which means that genetic and environmental factors interact in a complex way to determine who develops PA and who doesn't. In fact, we have known for a long time that a person has an increased susceptibility towards PA if there is family history of the disease. Recent advances in genetic technology have made it possible to explore these questions and we are now starting to identify the genes, changes in which cause PA in a handful of families.

There is still a long way to go before the genetics of pernicious anaemia are fully understood and he added this:

> However, we still do not know the genetic basis in a vast majority of individuals and families but I am confident that we will know much more about the genetics of PA in the coming years.

Dr Banka and his colleagues are continuing to make advances.

A gene called AIRE[iii] is essential for immune cells to recognise 'self'. It is, therefore, crucial in preventing autoimmunity. Recently, in a large collaborative study (Oftedal et al 2015), mutations were detected in the AIRE gene in many families with a range of organ-specific autoimmune conditions, including pernicious anaemia. Although the number of families in whom AIRE mutations would explain pernicious anaemia is small, it supports the long-held observation that genetic factors play a role in the development of pernicious anaemia. It also opens a new avenue for further research into the molecular basis of the disease. It is interesting that other conditions that can occur with AIRE mutations include Addison's disease, autoimmune thyroid disease and vitiligo.

I don't understand this whole genetics business (that's me talking, not Dr Banka) but I know that it is an exciting and growing field of science that holds out the promise of doctors being able to fully understand the nature of pernicious anaemia. Here's Dr Banka again:

Importantly, the genetic knowledge will improve our understanding of the disease which in turn could lead to better diagnosis, treatment and prevention of complications.

Pernicious anaemia and other conditions

Another strong indicator that a patient has pernicious anaemia, even though his/her test for intrinsic factor antibodies has returned as negative, is co-existing medical conditions. As we saw in Chapter 3, the range of medical conditions that can co-exist with pernicious

[iii] AIRE stands for Autoimmune Regulator.

anaemia is wide and various. Our own survey identified the following:

- depression (45%)
- tinnitus[iv] (34%)
- psoriasis, eczema or acne (28%)
- folic acid deficiency (23%)
- arrhythmia[v] (21%)
- hypothyroidism (19%)
- vitiligo (13%)
- rheumatoid arthritis (8%)
- diabetes mellitus (6%)
- coeliac disease (6%)
- previous *Helicobacter pylori* infection (5%)
- psoriatic arthritis (4%)
- hyperthyroidism (3%)
- hyperparathyroidism (1%)
- gastrectomy (1%)
- multiple sclerosis (0.2%)
- gastric cancer (0.1%).

Although our survey showed that 19% of patients whose low B$_{12}$ was caused by pernicious anaemia also suffered from hypothyroidism, in fact research has found that around 40% of patients with hypothyroidism also have a B$_{12}$ deficiency:

> There is a high (approx. 40%) prevalence of B12 deficiency in hypothyroid patients. Traditional symptoms are not a good guide to determining presence of B12 deficiency. Screening for vitamin B12 levels should be undertaken in all hypothyroid patients, irrespective of their thyroid antibody status. Replacement of B12 leads to improvement in symp-

[v] Tinnitus is characterised by screeching, whistling or ringing in the ears – sometimes all three at the same time.
[vi] Arrhythmia is the term for heartbeats that are irregular.

toms, although a placebo effect cannot be excluded, as a number of patients without B12 deficiency also appeared to respond to B12 administration.[5]

Depression was diagnosed in 45% of respondents but this high figure is most likely due to patients being told that they were suffering from depression when they asked for more frequent treatment (this happens far too often and will be discussed in the Chapters 5 and 6).

Now I'm not saying that doctors should be using co-existing conditions to diagnose pernicious anaemia; I'm not a doctor and it's not my place to tell medical professionals what they should or should not be doing. What I am saying is that perhaps modern physicians are not as aware as their predecessors of the link between pernicious anaemia and other (sometimes autoimmune) conditions, and that any of the above co-existing medical conditions might be used to raise suspicion that the patient might be suffering from pernicious anaemia. But there again, we know now that the test for pernicious anaemia is far from perfect and we are back at square one so to speak.

Autoimmune conditions

As we saw in Chapter 2, 'autoimmune metaplastic[vi] atrophic gastritis' is the underlying cause of pernicious anaemia. That first word, 'autoimmune', is used to describe a process whereby the body attacks itself for some reason or other – pernicious anaemia is a classic autoimmune disease because the body produces antibodies that destroy any intrinsic factor that has been produced. There are, as we have previously seen, a number of autoimmune diseases. Here's how the *Oxford Concise Dictionary of Medicine* defines autoimmune diseases:

[vi] Metaplastic refers to an abnormal change in tissue.

One of a number of otherwise unrelated disorders caused by inflammation and destruction of tissues by the body's own immune response. These disorders include acquired haemolytic anaemia, pernicious anaemia, rheumatic fever, rheumatoid arthritis, glomerulonephritis, systematic lupus erythematosus, myasthenia gravis, Sjögren's syndrome and several forms of thyroid dysfunction, including Hashimoto's disease.

And there are a lot more autoimmune conditions than those listed in the dictionary. They also include:

- alopecia areata – hair loss with typical patches of baldness
- autoimmune haemolytic anaemia – antibodies attack and burst red blood cells
- autoimmune hepatitis – the body's immune system attacks cells of the liver causing the liver to be inflamed
- dermatomyositis – inflammation of the muscles and skin
- diabetes (type 1) – a condition in which the immune system destroys insulin-producing cells of the pancreas, making it impossible for the body to use glucose (blood sugar) for energy; type 1 diabetes usually occurs in children and young adults
- some forms of juvenile idiopathic arthritis – inflamed, swollen and painful joints in young people
- glomerulonephritis – the immune system attacks tiny filters in the kidneys
- Graves' disease – an autoimmune disease of the thyroid gland that results in the overproduction of thyroid hormone; this causes such symptoms as nervousness, heat intolerance, heart palpitations and unexplained weight loss
- Guillain-Barré syndrome – the body's immune system attacks part of the nervous system, usually following a viral or bacterial infection
- immune thrombocytopenia – an attack on the blood's platelets
- some forms of myocarditis – inflammation of the heart muscle

- multiple sclerosis – the immune system believes the myelin sheath surrounding nerves is a foreign body and attacks it
- pemphigus/pemphigoid – autoantibodies attack the skin, usually around the groin
- polyarteritis nodosa – inflammation of the small and medium arteries
- polymyalgia rheumatic – inflammation of the muscles in the neck, shoulder and hip (generally); symptoms improve with exercise and are worst after rest
- polymyositis – inflammation of muscles
- primary biliary cirrhosis – damage to bile ducts in the liver
- psoriasis – a chronic skin disease that occurs when cells in the outer layer of the skin reproduce faster than normal
- psoriatic arthritis – a type of arthritis associated with psoriasis
- scleroderma/systemic sclerosis – hardening of the skin and sometimes internal organs
- some forms of uveitis – swelling of the middle area of the eye
- vitiligo – a disorder in which the immune system destroys pigment-making cells in the skin called melanocytes; this results in white patches of skin on different parts of the body
- granulomatosis with polyangiitis (Wegener's) – inflammation and swelling of the walls of blood vessels.

As with pernicious anaemia, the above conditions vary in their intensity, with the patient experiencing anything from mild to severe symptoms. There is also the fact that if a patient is unlucky enough to have one autoimmune disease the chances are he/she will have another or, unfortunately, several others. For example:

> Some patients also develop Hashimoto thyroiditis and 50% have thyroid antibodies; conversely, parietal cell antibodies are found in 30% of patients with thyroiditis.[6]

If autoimmune diseases were not enough to worry about, a great many patients are concerned that they are at a higher risk of developing gastric cancer than the general population. This causes a great deal of anxiety among some patients, who are frightened that they will develop stomach cancer – and this subject, along with psychiatric and neurological disorders, will be discussed at some length in Chapter 6 (see page 181).

Common mis-diagnoses

Given that there are such serious problems with firstly establishing the B$_{12}$ status of patients and then with the test to determine whether any deficiency is a consequence of pernicious anaemia, it shouldn't come as a surprise that patients are often told that the reason why they feel so ill is because they are suffering from some other disease or condition that might explain their symptoms. Our survey results show this to be the case. Before the final diagnosis of pernicious anaemia was made, respondents were asked if they were incorrectly given another explanation for their symptoms: 50% said 'no', 44% said 'yes' and the remaining 6% did not answer.

Now, even though it is to be expected that some mis-diagnoses will occur because of the problems with the tests involved, it really is quite astonishing that 44% of patients presenting to their doctor will have been told that their symptoms are due to something other than pernicious anaemia. According to our survey the most common mis-diagnoses were:

- anxiety and depression (16%)
- CFS/ME (5%)
- anaemia/iron deficiency (5%)
- irritable bowel syndrome (4%)
- underactive thyroid/hypothyroidism (4%)
- fibromyalgia (2.5%)
- multiple sclerosis (2.5%)

- hypochondria (2.5%)
- coeliac disease (2%)
- fatigue (1.5%)
- menopause (1.5%)
- diabetes (1%)
- post-viral fatigue (1%).

And there were numerous other explanations with less than 10 respondents identifying each.

It's easy to dismiss these figures as being of little significance, and indeed, some of the percentages are not large. However, there are two consequences that need to be understood. Firstly, whilst these percentages are not very large they should be seen against the large numbers of patients involved – around 3–5 million in the UK. Secondly, the figures don't reflect the associated unnecessary suffering, often for a good many years; nor do they tell the story of how careers, relationships, education and all manner of other aspects of everyday life are affected by the patients' suffering. This whole issue needs to be addressed and investigated by medical professionals in order to bring about a sea-change in how pernicious anaemia is diagnosed.

Chronic fatigue syndrome/ME and fibromyalgia

In our survey, 5% of patients were told that they were suffering from CFS/ME and 2.5% were told that fibromyalgia (FM) was the cause of their malaise. Given that the symptoms of these two conditions are similar and that the tests for B_{12} deficiency and pernicious anaemia are so problematic it is not surprising that doctors arrive at these (wrong) diagnoses. However, I would go one step further than this and suggest that a great many people who have been told that they have CFS/ME and fibromyalgia are actually suffering from a deficiency in vitamin B_{12}.

Now, you may be asking yourself what reasons do I have for making such a wild statement? And it's very simple. When patients with CFS/ME or fibromyalgia are given injections of vitamin B$_{12}$ they respond to this treatment almost immediately and see many of their symptoms disappear. Following on from a previous research programme which found that all 11 patients in the study with CFS and FM had elevated homocysteine levels (a reliable indicator of low B$_{12}$), a team of researchers from Gothenburg University in Sweden investigated whether patients responded to B$_{12}$ treatment and this is what they found:

> Frequent injections of high-concentrated vitamin B$_{12}$, combined with an individual daily dose of oral folic acid, may provide blood saturations high enough to be a remedy for good and safe relief in a subgroup of patients with ME/FM.[7]

Not all of the patients responded to the treatment in the same way and the research team believe that this could be due to other medicines interfering with the injections and with the MTHFR gene (which we'll look at in a tiny bit more detail soon – see page 129), but nevertheless they found that:

> Good responders rated themselves as 'very much' or 'much' improved, while Mild responders rated 'much' or 'minimally' improved.

Could these patients be suffering not from ME/FM but instead have undiagnosed pernicious anaemia? It's a valid hypothesis that really needs to be investigated more fully, and it leads to the question of just how many patients are suffering from the worst effects of ME and FM when all they need is injections of vitamin B$_{12}$?

Problems resulting from unclear test results

As will be clear from the discussion so far in this chapter, lack of diagnosis has a number of repercussions.

Firstly, there is always the danger that the patient's physician will attribute the patient's deficiency to a lack of B_{12} in his or her diet. This is not an unreasonable supposition if the doctor is unaware of the limitations of the intrinsic factor antibody test. The patient will be told to increase his or her intake of red meat and dairy, though I have yet to hear of any patient being told to eat raw offal – perhaps that's seen as unreasonable. The patient follows his or her doctor's instructions and sees no improvement in the symptoms, which will get progressively worse. And remember, there's now a very real possibility that the patient will develop serious and irreversible nerve damage, will underperform in the workplace and will often encounter problems at home. I know this because I have to deal with such issues on a regular basis.

The second consequence is that the patient will receive very little sympathy from family and friends, work colleagues and others who he or she might meet in the course of daily life. When you are suffering from the worst effects of B_{12} deficiency it is always helpful if you receive some recognition for the effort you have to make to get through normal daily life. Then there's the worry that accompanies a non-diagnosis. The patient worries that he or she is imagining the symptoms, or exaggerating them, and is left wondering if there will ever be an improvement in how he or she feels – and this worrying never goes away.

Thirdly there is the problem that, even if the physician will sanction treatment by prescribing injections, there is every likelihood that treatment will be stopped when the patient's serum B_{12} becomes elevated. Patients with a diagnosis of pernicious anaemia have the security that their injections will be for life and will never be stopped. (Well, in an ideal world this would be the case, but patients having their treatment terminated are not unheard of even if they have been diagnosed as having pernicious anaemia.)

You may be one of the unfortunate patients who has all of the classical symptoms of B$_{12}$ deficiency but has not received a definitive explanation of why you are deficient. Perhaps you know somebody who is unwell, has a family history of pernicious anaemia but hasn't tested positive for intrinsic factor antibodies and consequently remains undiagnosed.

The options open to people in these situations are either to bypass their doctor and begin to self-medicate, either with or without their physician's consent or knowledge, or, simply to continue to suffer the symptoms of the deficiency, which can and does lead to severe, irreversible nerve damage.

The survey of members of the Pernicious Anaemia Society shows that at diagnosis only 32% of patients underwent the test for serum intrinsic factor antibodies and only 14% the test for serum parietal cell antibodies. Could this be because primary care doctors realise the limitations of the tests?

Bella's story

I like to think that I've become 'case hardened' over the years to the way in which some patients are treated, or, in the case of 15-year-old Bella Rockchick (not her real name, you understand), not treated.

It was Bella's mother who first made contact with the Society's office. I don't have a full transcript of the phone conversation but she told me that her 15-year-old daughter had been ill for years suffering from the symptoms of severe B$_{12}$ deficiency.

'She's continually tired, attends school only for a few hours in the morning, then comes home and sleeps for six hours – more if I don't wake her.

'She has problems with her concentration and memory, she's irritable, has severe sudden mood swings and because of all this she doesn't have a social life at all.'

It was a tale that I had heard before and of course, as I mentioned in my first book *Pernicious Anaemia: the forgotten disease*, it is the tale of teenagers with pernicious anaemia that I find most frustrating and which sadden me most. However, it's what Bella's mother went on to say that really worried me.

'Now she's having problems walking, her hands and feet are extremely painful and she's getting pins and needles.

'We managed to get her doctor to give her an injection of B_{12} every week for a month over Christmas and we couldn't believe the difference in her – we even caught her smiling for the first time in years,' she said.

It was at this point that I suggested that she and her daughter come to see me so that they could discuss the options available to them. They duly arrived at the offices of the Pernicious Anaemia Society after a three-hour car journey. What I saw startled me, but I have learned that rather than getting angry it is best to channel my energy into bringing about change in the way in which pernicious anaemia is diagnosed and treated – and this change will only come about by exerting pressure on those in authority to conduct a thorough review of the current issues associated with the disease.

Bella was a pretty young girl who was slightly built. As she walked towards me I was reminded how I walked immediately before my diagnosis - just like Herman Munster or an early portrayal of Frankenstein in films. My heart sank; what kind of future lay ahead for this young lady? What could I do about it?

Bella and her mother and father began to tell their sad tale; how this deterioration had been going on for years; how doctors didn't seem to believe them; how a few pennies' worth of injections had turned her outlook around and how they felt right now – helpless; and how her B$_{12}$ levels were borderline but that she had tested negative for the intrinsic factor antibodies. I was glad I was able to help them to understand what their daughter was going through – I ended up with permanent nerve damage and a Herman Munster walk. I suggested that they print out the bulletin of the new guidelines from the Library section of the Society's website and hand it to Bella's doctor: 'We've done that – he wouldn't read them.'

We discussed over-the-counter remedies, including the new sub-lingual spray which interested them, as they had been using it, though only sparingly. And it was then that I told them about doctors whose practice includes intravenous infusions of methylcobalamin and self-injecting sub-cutaneous methylcobalamin as often as the patient sees fit. That was when I could see that Bella's parents had, for the first time in many years, some hope of dealing with their daughter's problems. I provided them with the names of a few doctors near them who would be able to help and they left the office a lot happier than when they had first arrived. I couldn't be sure, but as Bella shuffled away I thought she had a slight spring in her step.

Summary

In this chapter we have seen that it is now acknowledged that the test to determine whether a patient's low B_{12} status is due to pernicious anaemia is seriously flawed, and is not identifying all patients with classic pernicious anaemia. Furthermore, according to the new BCSH guidelines, even if a patient tests negative for intrinsic factor antibodies, he or she could still have pernicious anaemia. We also know that doctors are reluctant to give a firm diagnosis of pernicious anaemia without a positive result for the antibodies. All of the above means that there is a growing number of patients who might have been identified as being deficient in B_{12} but who are not told the reason for that deficiency. Instead, the physician may attribute the deficiency to diet and will often tell the patient to eat more red meat and return in six months or so to have his/her B_{12} status reassessed.

You might now be beginning to appreciate why, when telephone callers to the Pernicious Anaemia Society's office tell me they have just been diagnosed as having pernicious anaemia, my first reaction is often to congratulate them; I'm not being facetious or trying to be clever in any way. I'm genuinely glad that the patient has received a firm diagnosis and is not one of the many who are B_{12} deficient but whose test for pernicious anaemia was negative and who live in a sort of twilight world of not being told why they feel so ill. And with that in mind, it's time to look at how pernicious anaemia is treated. Don't think that this will be plain sailing either.

References

1 Landl JH. *William B Castle, 1887–1990: A Biographical Memoir.* Washington DC: National Academy of Science; 1995.

2 http://www.nasonline.org/publications/biographical-memoirs/memoir-pdfs/castle-wb.pdf (Accessed 24 February2015).

3 Ibid.

4 Khan S, , Del-Duca C, Fenton E, Holding S, Hirst J, Doré PC, Sewell WA. Limited value of testing for intrinsic factor antibodies with negative gastric parietal cell antibodies in pernicious anaemia. *Journal of Clinical Pathology* 2009; 62:439–441.

5 Oftedal BE, Hellesen A, Erichsen MM, Bratland E, Vardi A, Perheentupa J, Kemp EH, Fiskerstrand T, Viken MK, Weetman AP, Fleishman SJ, Banka S, Newman WG, Sewell WA, Sozaeva LS, Zayats T, Haugarvoll K, Orlova EM, Haavik J, Johansson S, Knappskog PM, Løvås K, Wolff AS, Abramson J, Husebye ES. Dominant mutations in the autoimmune regulator AIRE are associated with common organ-specific autoimmune diseases. *Immunity* 2015; 16;42(6):1185-1967.

6 Devalia V, Hamilton MS, Molloy A-M. Guidelines for the diagnosis and treatment of cobalamin and folate disorders. *British Journal of Haematology* 2014; 166(4):496–513.

7 Jabbar A, Yawar A, Waseem S, Islam N, Ul Haque N, Zuberi L, Khan A, Akhter J. Vitamin B$_{12}$ deficiency common in primary hypothyroidism. *Journal of Pakistan Medical Association* 2008; 58(5):258–261.

8 DiMarino MC. Autoimmune metaplastic atrophic gastritis. *Merck Manual 2014.* http://www.merckmanuals.com/professional/gastro-intestinal-disorders/gastritis-and-peptic-ulcer-disease/autoimmune-metaplastic-atrophic-gastritis (Accessed 15 April 2015).

9 Regland B. Forsmark S, Halaouate L, Matousek M, Peilot B, Zachrisson O, et al. Response to Vitamin B$_{12}$ and Folic Acid in Myalgic Encephalomyelitis and Fibromyalgia. *PLoS ONE* 2015; 10(4): doi: 10.1371/journal.pone.0124648

Chapter 5

Problems with the treatment of pernicious anaemia

The road to patients receiving a firm diagnosis of pernicious anaemia is, as we have seen, often a long and tortuous one, so you would expect that when a patient is eventually told why he or she feels so poorly, the treatment would be a pretty straightforward affair – but often it isn't. In fact, the way in which patients are currently treated is by far the biggest cause of complaint by members of the Pernicious Anaemia Society. However, before we start looking at the issue of inadequate treatment I have to deal with the grim reality that sometimes the patient isn't treated at all.

Refusal of treatment

I have heard at first hand from a handful of patients who, when they received their diagnosis, were simply told that they should change their diet, eat more red meat and return in six months' time to have their serum B_{12} checked again. Thankfully these instances are rare, but they do occur. My advice to the patient is to simply make an appointment with another doctor at the practice or, if this is not possible, to tell the doctor concerned that he or she has contacted the Pernicious Anaemia Society who are 'extremely concerned'. That is usually enough for the wayward doctor to commence treatment.

However, a much more frequent situation is treatment being stopped after initial diagnosis and commencement of injections. This usually happens following a routine blood test which shows that the patient's B$_{12}$ level is high. This leads doctors to withdraw treatment until the patient's blood returns to normal (whatever that is). The simple fact is that any patient receiving replacement therapy injections of B$_{12}$ will have high levels of B$_{12}$ in their blood – all it proves is that the injections are getting through and doing what they are supposed to do. The explanation given for the cessation of the patient's treatment is often, though not always, accompanied by some quite bizarre statements that would be laughable if they didn't cause so much confusion and distress among patients. For example, 'your blood will thicken'; 'your liver will fail'; 'your heart will not be able to cope with all that B$_{12}$'; 'high levels of B$_{12}$ are extremely dangerous'.

And it is not only doctors who are responsible for stopping patients' treatment. Nurses are also guilty of failing to realise that patients who are receiving B$_{12}$ injections will have high serum levels of the vitamin if their treatment is working properly. Put simply, it is not possible to monitor the serum B$_{12}$ status of patients for 'normality' once injections have begun as the level should always be high. There is an anomaly to all this, however: some patients will have low, or lower than expected, levels of B$_{12}$ in the run-up to their next injection, which is often cited as evidence that they need more frequent injections. Why this is so has, as far as I'm aware, never been investigated. Anyway, the new British Committee for Standards in Haematology (BCSH) guidelines make a very good point – once a patient has received a diagnosis of having pernicious anaemia they should never have their treatment stopped:

> Patients suspected of having pernicious anaemia should be tested for IFAB. Patients found to be positive should have *lifelong* therapy with cobalamin.

Unfortunately, some patients are told that because they have reached a certain age they no longer require any further injections. One member of the Pernicious Anaemia Society is a manager of a nursing home in South Wales. A few years ago he attended the opening of the new office of the Society and told the MP who was performing the ceremony that the previous week six of his residents, all over the age of 80, had been told by the community nurse who visited the home to administer the injections that they no longer needed them. The manager immediately telephoned the medical centre to express his horror at his residents' treatment and the doctor duly authorised them to continue. It helped that the manager himself had pernicious anaemia and knew that injections are needed for life – if he hadn't had personal experience of the disease perhaps the outcome would have been different.

Only this week (as I write) I had a telephone call from a lady aged 80 who had received a firm diagnosis of pernicious anaemia 20 years earlier and whose injections had then been stopped five years ago. She could no longer walk and asked if I could telephone her GP's Practice Manager to find out what was going on. I spoke to the Practice Manager and sent a copy of the new BCSH guidelines. The next day the patient called me to tell me one of the GPs had telephoned her and arranged for a Community Nurse to inject her later that morning. I then telephoned the surgery again and requested that the patient receive 'loading doses' of B_{12} every other day until the neurological issues improved no further. This time I spoke to a GP who also requested a copy of the guidelines.

Frequency of treatment

Cessation, or refusal, of treatment is not, however, the major cause of concern amongst patients, as thankfully most doctors are aware that replacement therapy injections must take place for the lifetime of the patient. Unfortunately, the biggest cause of concern is the frequency with which injections are given. Given that complaints about the way in which patients who have pernicious anaemia are treated are so widespread, it is disappointing that the new BCSH guidelines say very little about this whole issue. Instead they refer physicians to the *British National Formulary* (BNF),[i] which sets out the guidance for the treatment of patients. Here's what the BCSH say:

> Current clinical practice within the UK is to treat cobalamin deficiency with hydroxocobalamin in the intramuscular form (outlined in the *British National Formulary*).

The guidelines then go on to quote the *BNF*:

> Standard initial therapy for patients without neurological involvement is 1000 mcg intramuscularly (i.m.) three times a week for 2 weeks. The BNF advises that patients presenting with neurological symptoms should receive 1000 mcg i.m. on alternate days until there is no further improvement.

There are two things to note here. Firstly, newly diagnosed patients should receive what are known as 'loading doses' for two weeks – that's three injections a week for two weeks. Unfortunately, not all patients receive these loading doses. Secondly, if the patient has any neurological symptoms (numbness, pins and needles, unusual gait, balance problems etc), then injections must be given every other day 'until there is no further improvement'. Unfortunately, this also often does not happen.

However, the guidelines then go on to challenge the *BNF* by stating that the BCSH cannot see any point in giving injections every other day for longer than three weeks and not, as the *BNF* says, 'until there

---

[i] The *BNF* is published by the Royal Pharmaceutical Society and the British Medical Association. It describes what medicines are to be used to treat particular medical conditions and diseases.

is no further improvement':

> However, the GWG[ii] recommends a pragmatic approach in
> patients with neurological symptoms by reviewing the need
> for continuation of alternate day therapy after 3 weeks of
> treatment.

Now, lots of commentators on social media sites are highly critical of this, believing that the new guidelines mean that patients with neurological issues will stop receiving injections every other day once they have had three weeks' worth. That is not, however, what the new guidelines state – they recommend a 'pragmatic approach' and suggest that the physician and the patient 'review' the need for such frequent injections simply because they assume that if the patient was going to show any improvement in neurological symptoms, then he or she would do so within three weeks.

As an illustration of why such a review may be necessary, I took a telephone call recently from a lady who had neurological involvement who asked when she should expect to feel any improvement in her condition. I asked how long she had been receiving injections every other day and her reply startled me – 'Two and a half years,' she said. I had to break the bad news to her that if she had been receiving such intensive treatment for so long it was highly unlikely that she would feel any further improvement now, but then suggested that she should discuss this with her doctor as perhaps there was no point in her continuing with injections every other day. Her response startled me further: 'Oh, I'm so glad to hear that. It takes up so much time and my arms are continually aching from the injections.'

As we have seen, the Pernicious Anaemia Society's survey found that, 'when asked if they were satisfied with their treatment, 64% said "No", 28% said "Yes" and the remaining 8% did not provide an answer.'

[ii] Guidelines Writing Group.

Those figures have to be seen in context – some of those who said yes will be self-medicating and bypassing their doctor. The 64% who said they were not satisfied with their treatment would probably have been higher if those who are self-medicating had been excluded. And of course, in certain cases, the patient's doctor will readily sanction more frequent injections, though this doesn't happen as often as it should.

There's something else that needs to be borne in mind – these figures are a quantifiable reflection of the many debates and posts on various social media where the question of treatment is the most common topic of debate. While 64% may be a lower proportion than perhaps it should be, it still remains the case that two-thirds of the patients in the survey were not satisfied with the treatment that they were receiving. And the survey went further and asked respondents to choose a word that best described how they rated their medical care. The results were:

- very poor (20%)
- inadequate (18%)
- good (10%)
- poor (10%)
- undecided (9%)
- reasonable (8%)
- adequate (8%)
- very good (7%)
- excellent (3%)
- unreasonable (2%).

(The remaining 5% of respondents did not answer the question.)

You can see that a large number of patients were dissatisfied with their treatment: half reported it as being poor, very poor, inadequate or unreasonable. Whilst 10% of patients considered their treatment as being 'very good' or 'excellent', the survey results demonstrate that many patients are unhappy with the standard of treatment they receive in the UK, with the consequence that an increasing number of patients seek alternative sources of B_{12} and self-treat, sometimes with the consent and knowledge of their doctor but most often without. The academic paper based on our survey commented:

> According to personal observations by the lead author, patients who are unhappy with current NHS treatment increasingly seek alternative sources of vitamin B_{12}. As well as intravenous infusions, which make up the most common delivery method, other modes of delivery include sublingual sprays and drops as well as skin patches and nasal sprays. Patients who are unable to convince their doctor that they need more frequent injections than the one usually pre-scribed every 12 weeks in the UK increasingly resort to such alternatives. This has been driven by the many social media sites found on the internet and by manufacturers reacting to a demand for self-administered treatments. No thorough investigation into their efficacy has been carried out. Most new products use methyl-B_{12}, although it is not licensed for use in the UK. Of the survey respondents, 10% reported using methyl-B12 to either replace or supplement their prescribed injections.

I now realise that I was fortunate when I was eventually diagnosed as having pernicious anaemia in being allowed an injection every three weeks. Most UK doctors will not prescribe more frequent injections than one every three months even though the patient presents a good case for having one earlier. The worst case of in-transigence by a medical professional that I have come across was when a member of the Pernicious Anaemia Society telephoned with the following experience. This lady was middle-aged and had for many years endured (unnecessary) suffering through having to wait three months for her next injection. She told me that as 'regular as clockwork' she felt a return of her symptoms five weeks after her injection; she struggled to cope with her work and home life for the remaining period until she was allowed another. She then told me what had happened when she took a two-week holiday with her family. She had been looking forward to this but it was due to begin half-way through the twelfth week after her previous injection; she therefore turned up at her doctor's surgery for her next injection just a few days early, knowing this would mean she would be able to enjoy her two weeks' break. The nurse, however, refused and that meant that, in her words, she 'had the most miserable two weeks of my life'. As soon as she was back home she went straight to the nurse to receive her injection but the holiday had been wasted.

It's not all gloom and doom. Some doctors are more than willing to depart from the *BNF* guidelines. And now it's time to introduce you to Grumpy Git – the self-imposed sobriquet of Roy Sandiford, a long-time member of the Pernicious Anaemia Society. Grumpy Git (this is, you have to understand, his preferred name) underwent an ileostomy many years ago and has fought for years to get replacement therapy injections based on his needs. After battling for many years to get a prescription for an injection every four weeks he moved house and had to embark on another battle to get adequate treatment from his new local surgery. His story gives some hope for the great many sufferers who need more frequent injections. This is what he sent me in an email:

> To remind you of my condition, I am an Ileostomist and the best previous treatment by various GPs, had been four-weekly injections. I changed GP practice yet again in March 2014, where the nurse I was interviewed by offered to up-grade injections of B12 from four weekly to two weekly. As is 'normal' these days, one of the GPs of the practice immediately over-ruled the new routine, reprimanding the nurse for over-stepping her position. Being the type of person my

email name suggests, I then went to the senior doctor of the practice who checked the details of my complaint with me. Dr C then immediately agreed to me going on to *two-weekly* jabs. He arranged for me to have an injection immediately. Two weeks later, before my injection, the nurse did another blood test. A few days later I received a phone call to say my levels were *just* over the top of the standard level used and did I wish to continue with two-weekly, or reduce them.
I opted to continue and am still on *two-weekly injections.* FEELING MUCH BETTER.

I can almost hear people saying 'lucky Grumpy Git' as they read this.

How on earth did things get so bad? Why is there so much dissatisfaction among patients with their treatment, which is, we should remind ourselves, a simple vitamin supplementation? In order to answer these questions we need to go back in history to see how things have developed the way they have.

History of pernicious anaemia treatment

For nearly 100 years following the identification of pernicious anaemia as a medical condition, patients received no effective treatment. Their disease would mean that they would undergo a long and gradual demise, perhaps free of pain but not without a great deal of discomfort. Doctors were helpless to halt the gradual deterioration in the patient and could only look on, along with the patient's family and friends, as his or her condition deteriorated. In the 1920s it was discovered that feeding patients large doses of, preferably raw, liver could keep them alive and it's a tribute to human ingenuity that before long raw or slightly cooked liver was being given to patients in liquid form and various other ways – liver soup is, apparently, quite edible if laced with brandy. (Some people still use raw chicken livers in breakfast smoothies.)

By the late 1940s various pharmaceutical companies were producing 'liver extract injections' whereby concentrated liver preparations were being injected directly into the patient's body. During the late 1940s the first artificially produced B_{12} injections were made available, and it was around this time that doctors became concerned with just how much of the newly available artificially produced B_{12} should be given to patients in order for them not only to be kept alive but also, hopefully, to lead a normal life. And it was this attempt to identify what would constitute an adequate treatment regime that has led to by far the largest complaint by members of the Pernicious Anaemia Society – the inadequacy of the treatment that they receive. To find out why the issue of treatment of pernicious anaemia is such a contentious issue we have to go back to those days immediately following the end of the Second World War.

As stated, between the mid-1920s and late-1940s, the way in which patients with pernicious anaemia were kept alive was by feeding them raw or slightly cooked liver. Nobody really worried about the amount that the patient ingested; the only worry would have been centred on whether the patient was actually taking his or her 'medicine'. Recipes of the time suggested various combinations of ingredients and usually featured offal of some type or other. But whilst the recipes did mention how much of the offal should be included, it was probably because the amount stated would have the taste best camouflaged by the other ingredients. Nobody worried about overdosing on the amount of offal ingested, rather there would have been relief that the patient was actually consuming the food and adhering to the new diet.

Now, you may be wondering why an offal-heavy diet would have kept people with pernicious anaemia alive when we know that this group of patients were unable to extract vitamin B_{12} from food because they lacked the necessary intrinsic factor. The reason is the same as why some patients today prefer to take tablets of B_{12} rather than receive injections – some of the B_{12} tablet, just as some of the offal, *will* be absorbed in the ileum even without any intrinsic factor being present.

Remember, we saw that a normal healthy human will have in their stomach a substance called intrinsic factor and that the intrinsic factor will bind to any B_{12} swallowed as food and will make its way to the last section of the small intestine, the ileum, where it will pass through the lining of the ileum and into the bloodstream. If the patient doesn't have any of the intrinsic factor in his or her stomach, then he or she won't be able to transport the B_{12}/intrinsic factor mixture into the ileum, where it would be transferred into the bloodstream, right? Well, yes and no.

You see, if a patient swallows large amounts of foodstuffs containing B_{12}, or swallows a tablet containing a large dose of B_{12}, the B_{12} will find its way into the ileum without any intrinsic factor binding to it and, once in the ileum, a small amount will be absorbed into the bloodstream 'passively' – it's a process that doctors call 'passive infusion': 'About 1% of large oral doses of vitamin B_{12} passively diffuses into the bloodstream from the small intestine.'[1] That's why those patients from the mid-1920s were able to be kept alive – they ingested large amounts of B_{12} in the form of offal and then sat back with their fingers crossed and hoped that some of the vitamin would get into their bloodstream.

And the same thing happens nowadays when patients use high-dosage tablets to correct their deficiency – taking a full 1 mg of B_{12} in tablet form will mean that some of it, or rather *hopefully* some of it, will be absorbed 'passively' in the ileum. I'll examine the debate about the efficacy of oral versus parenteral[iii] treatment later in this chapter (page 145). Anyway, by the late 1940s, as I have said previously, various

---

iii Parenteral means injected.

pharmaceutical companies were producing concentrated liver extract injections which were being used to treat pernicious anaemia, and, soon after, artificial B$_{12}$ was being produced, although this was initially on a small scale.

It then became obvious that an optimum treatment regimen needed to be identified and a protocol based on these injections was needed. Doctors began asking how much of the new injectable B$_{12}$ was needed to correct a patient's deficiency. Until this time, doctors had been content to just inject patients with various amounts of liver extract, satisfied with the knowledge that given enough of the therapy the patient would stay alive. But why did doctors suddenly want to know how much and how regularly the patient would need the new artificial B$_{12}$ injections? Surely if the injections worked and there was no danger of the patient overdosing on B$_{12}$, no specific protocol was needed?

I haven't been able to find a definitive answer to that question but I suggest that it could be due to two reasons. Firstly, doctors are scientists and they like to work with scientific protocols and guidelines based on established data. Secondly, the injections would have been expensive (more expensive than raw ox liver at any rate), and so it would have been economic as well as scientifically judicious to lay down an established treatment regime in a protocol that other doctors could follow. And what happens next is nothing short of jaw-dropping.

US research 1948–1958

Now here's something to ponder. Imagine you were asked to investigate how much B$_{12}$ patients with pernicious anaemia would need to allow them (a) to live and (b) to enjoy a normal life. One hundred milligrams per day? Five hundred milligrams per week? A few thousand milligrams per year? Well, this is one of the questions that a group of doctors were asking themselves when, in 1948 – just a year after B_{12} had been identified – they started out on a 10-year investigation into how much and how often the new B_{12} injections should be administered to patients.

Their conclusions wouldn't just establish a treatment protocol that other doctors would follow, but would also provide the basis for the establishment of the nutritional requirements for people who did not have pernicious anaemia. Obviously, the more patients that were involved in the experiment the more accurate would be the results. However, the fact is that the entire vitamin B_{12} treatment protocol for patients with pernicious anaemia for the European Union, the USA, Canada and the Nordic countries is based on a study that began in 1948 using just *seven* people. That isn't a misprint. All seven patients had been diagnosed as having pernicious anaemia and they were all experiencing a return of their symptoms.[2]

The team of doctors that took it upon themselves to find out just how much B_{12} was needed and how often it was to be delivered was based in Nashville, Tennessee, in the United States, and was led by William J Darby, MD. It was an international collaboration involving doctors from Brazil and Guatemala, although all of the patients were from Nashville. It was a remarkable investigation because the investigators numbered eight – one person more than the number of patients they were studying. Now you'd think that the actual methodology would be straightforward – the doctors would give the patients injections of various amounts of B_{12}, measure their serum B_{12} and keep measuring it until it dropped below a certain numerical indicator and then give another injection. However, there was a problem – in those days they were unable to measure a patient's B_{12} – there was no 'marker' for B_{12} available to them. (A 'marker' in this sense means a biomarker or biological marker which is a measurable indicator of a biological state or condition – in this case an indicator of B_{12} status.) A subsequent researcher comments:

Notably, that study used haematological status for health

characterization, and not vitamin B-12 biomarkers because the major portion of the data was obtained prior to the existence of suitable methods for measuring them.[3]

The haematological indicators used by the researchers were packed cell volume (PCV) and mean corpuscular volume (MCV) of the patients' blood.

- PCV is a way of measuring a patient's *haematocrit* – the number of red blood cells in a given amount of blood. A normal healthy person will have around 40% of their blood made up of red blood cells.
- MCV measures the size of the red blood cells. Oversized red blood cells are known as macrocytic cells; smaller than average red blood cells are known as microcytic; and normal-sized red blood cells are known as normocytic. As we have noted in earlier chapters, enlarged red blood cells are an indicator of B12 deficiency (though not in all cases) while small red blood cells are an indicator of iron deficiency.

It was by using these haematological indicators that the doctors began their 10-year investigation into how much B₁₂ an average person needed. After reading this I decided to do a little more investigation and managed to get hold of the original paper that was published in 1958. The doctors published their paper in the *American Journal of Medicine*[4] and it has, among all the figures and tables, some remarkable findings that could go some way to explaining why so many patients with pernicious anaemia are unhappy with their treatment. Here's what the authors had to say:

> No greater effect was detected in one instance by increasing the dose above 0.5 mcg, in two by increasing it from 1.0 to 2.0 mcg, or in two by increasing it from 2.0 to 4.0 mcg. In only one instance was an increase above 2.0 mcg daily followed by a detectable change.

What they are saying here is that some patients managed perfectly well on 0.5 mcg while others needed 2 mcg – in other words, different patients need different amounts of B_{12} daily.

Again, in their conclusion they note that: 'The minimal daily dietary needs for this vitamin may be met by approximately 0.6 to 2.8 mcg with a narrower range of 0.6 to 1.2 mcg. sufficient for most persons' – note that they say 'most persons' and not all persons. They continue: 'It seems justifiable to conclude, therefore, that maintenance of maximal erythropoiesis requires the daily utilization of from 0.5 to 2.0 mcg of vitamin B_{12}. In most subjects the quantity appears to be between 0.5 and 1.0 mcg'; that means that some people need four times the daily amount of B_{12} than others. And there's one more little quote I want to share with you: 'The patients who exhibited good initial response to the smallest dosages were those who required the least quantities for maintenance and vice versa.'

In other words, the patients who were given large doses initially needed large doses for maintenance, while those who were started off on small doses only needed small doses in the future. Now why could that be? Often when modern-day patients ask for more frequent injections they are told that 'the more you receive the more you want' which, as far as I've been able to discover is based on no scientific evidence, but is a way of telling the patient that he or she is imagining that they need more injections. But the 1958 paper was not based on patient's feeling of wellbeing but instead on close inspection of the patient's blood. And patients who were given large doses initially needed large doses for maintenance, not to feel well but to prevent their blood deteriorating. Why this was the case is not explained by the researchers and I haven't been able to find any papers that re-examine this phenomenon.

To sum up then, the researchers in the 1940s and 1950s on whose findings the daily requirements of B_{12} in humans is based state quite clearly that different people need different amounts. Today patients with pernicious anaemia are prescribed a one-size-fits-all treatment regimen, or at least that's the case in the UK. Could the fact that they, the patients, are not able to receive treatment based on their needs be the reason why there is so much dissatisfaction with their treatment that leads them to bypass their doctor and source further treatment themselves?

Before we leave 1958 behind there's something else that needs to be said – those recommendations about B$_{12}$ intake are for *daily* requirements. Normal healthy individuals will not need to take a 2 mcg tablet of B$_{12}$ every day to ensure that they don't become deficient, unless they are strict vegans. Eating a balanced diet which includes meat, fish and dairy products will ensure that a healthy individual will not become deficient in B$_{12}$ and you don't need to go out of your way to ensure that you are getting adequate amounts of B$_{12}$ – drinking a cup of milky coffee with your breakfast of bacon and eggs will provide you with a decent hit of B$_{12}$, and throughout the day, ordinary food and drink will provide the rest of your daily requirement. In contrast, patients with pernicious anaemia are given a large dose of B$_{12}$ every three months, and it is assumed that they will be able to store the vitamin in and around their liver to ensure that they will be able to make healthy red blood cells for the next 12 weeks. Wouldn't it be much better if patients were treated like normal, healthy individuals and given small, but adequate, doses of B$_{12}$ that bypassed the stomach on a daily basis? Of course it would, and there are moves towards this becoming a reality – more of this in Chapter 8 (page 217).

Before leaving our historical survey of pernicious anaemia treatments, there is one other suggestion to consider. Wouldn't it be even more effective to address the underlying cause of the B$_{12}$ deficiency in patients with pernicious anaemia: the lack of intrinsic factor? You see, all this talk of replacement therapy injections has led me to think 'outside the box' and to consider that the answer to all of my ills lies not with artificially produced B_{12} but with intrinsic factor. Surely it would be smiles all around if I could be given some intrinsic factor which would mean that I - and my fellow pernicious anaemia sufferers - would be able to eat a balanced diet and receive all of the B_{12} I needed from food? I thought I had stumbled on the ideal solution to the problems posed by pernicious anaemia – give patients intrinsic factor and let the patient's body do the rest. I even tested my hypothesis on Dr Ralph Carmel. Unfortunately, my solution was not the revelation I had hoped it would have been. Dr Carmel said, 'Oral doses of intrinsic factor were tried in Europe about 50 years ago, but many patients eventually developed antibodies to the animal intrinsic factor and became refractory to it.'

Oh well, it was worth a go I suppose, but somebody had already thought of it. So it's back to the problem with patients getting treatment according to their need.

Methods of treatment

Oral tablets versus injections

Now, if there's one topic that is guaranteed to annoy patients with pernicious anaemia, it's the subject of oral supplementation. In some parts of the world patients are having their deficiency treated by oral tablets because, as was discussed earlier, it has been proved that around 1% of ingested B_{12} will be absorbed in the ileum by what is known as 'passive diffusion'. If a person with pernicious anaemia takes a whopping dose of B_{12} in tablet form some of the B_{12} will be absorbed, or, maybe more accurately some of the B_{12} should be absorbed by passive diffusion.

Experiments have shown that this is the case, and it must work because I know that some patients have opted for this method of treatment –

usually because they are totally needle-phobic. A Cochrane review[iv] showed that: 'High oral doses of B$_{12}$ (1000 mcg and 2000 mcg) were as effective as intramuscular administration in achieving haematological and neurological responses.'[5]

And the authors go on to explain that: 'The evidence derived from these limited studies suggests that 2000 mcg doses of oral vitamin B$_{12}$ daily and 1000 mcg doses initially daily and thereafter weekly and then monthly may be as effective as intramuscular administration in obtaining short-term haematological and neurological responses in vitamin B$_{12}$ deficient patients.'

All is not as clear cut as it first appears, however. Notice that they use the word 'may' when they talk of the effectiveness of the tablets and they are talking of 'short-term' responses. The review was based on studies that were not really fully representative of patients with pernicious anaemia and this is reflected in the Pernicious Anaemia Society's Policy on cyanocobalamin tablets, which calls for more research to take place into the efficacy of tablets before any attempt is made to introduce oral supplementation instead of injections. And it's not only patients who are suspicious of the use of tablets as B$_{12}$ replacement therapy; in countries where tablets have been introduced as the preferred method of treating the consequences of pernicious anaemia, there is evidence that doctors continue to pre-scribe injections – perhaps because they realise that the patients will simply resort to buying injectable B$_{12}$ from other sources, including the internet.

Patients in the UK who choose oral tablets over injections are forced to purchase 1 mg tablets from internet stores, because at the time of writing 1 mg tablets are not available on prescription, though 50 mcg tablets of cyanocobalamin are. It's just another example of how

---

[iv] The Cochrane Collaboration undertakes systematic reviews of all relevant randomised controlled trials of health care.

patients with pernicious anaemia lack any real choice relating to their treatment. The good news is that 1 mg tablets cost as little as three pence from internet stores.

The authors of the new BCSH guidelines are not great fans of oral treatment in pernicious anaemia, which can be seen as an indicator that injections are not going to be phased out any time soon. Here's what they say:

> High dose oral cyanocobalamin (1000–2000 mcg) is licensed for use in several countries outside the UK and is widely available via the internet. Passive, intrinsic factor-independent absorption of a small fraction of such large doses *should* suffice to meet daily requirements.[v]

The guidelines then go on to mention the Cochrane review I mentioned above, before adding a note of caution:

> However, the efficacy and cost-effectiveness of oral treatment in wider population-based settings has yet to be established. There are arguments against the use of oral cobalamin in initiation of cobalamin therapy in severely deficient individuals who have poor absorption, especially due to pernicious anaemia.

The guidelines also state that:

> High dose oral cobalamin would be a reasonable alternative as maintenance in patients unable to tolerate intramuscular injections provided there is good compliance with treatment.

Let's get one thing straight – intramuscular Injections are not pleasant. They need to be administered by a trained medical professional who, hopefully, is able to take his or her time when carrying out the

---

[v] My emphasis.

procedure – and that includes letting the solution warm to room temperature before injecting as cold hydroxocobalamin is thick and does not inject easily. So why do so many patients prefer these time-consuming, often painful injections over simply popping a pill every day? I wouldn't want to take pills instead of my injections for one very good reason. It has been explained to me that I am unable to absorb B$_{12}$ from food because I lack intrinsic factor. And it has also been explained to me that if I take a large dose of B$_{12}$ daily then around 1% *may* be absorbed by passive infusion. That word '*may*' troubles me. I know how I felt when I was eventually diagnosed, and I'm sorry but I am not going to take a chance on me going back to how I was then if I don't happen to be able to passively diffuse oral B$_{12}$. Unlike people who don't have pernicious anaemia, if I was to resort to oral supplementation then, as I swallowed the tablet, I would have my fingers firmly crossed that I would absorb some of the B$_{12}$ I was swallowing. I simply don't want to take that chance and this is something that the new guidelines address: 'On the other hand, some patients may prefer intramuscular injection therapy in order to assure effective treatment' – Exactly!

Just before Christmas 2014 I received a telephone call from one of our members from the south-west of England. She told me that she, presumably along with other patients with pernicious anaemia at her health centre, had received a letter stating that because of new scientific developments she would no longer have to suffer the inconvenience of visiting the surgery every three months to receive her injection because new research had shown that 1 mg tablets of B$_{12}$ are as effective at treating her condition as injections. The letter also stated that unfortunately the 1 mg tablets were not available via the NHS but could be readily obtained from Amazon and health food stores.

More alarming was the statement that this move towards oral tablets was endorsed by the Pernicious Anaemia Society – which was quite untrue. The member was telephoning to verify that we, as a Society, were in favour of this move which, of course, we were not. I immediately telephoned the Practice Manager concerned. It was New Year's Eve when the doctor did telephone with an apology, saying he had recently been on a training day and he must have misinterpreted what had been said. He promised to write another letter to all of the patients who had received the original letter and ask them to make an appointment to discuss this issue with their doctor. He also agreed to retract the statement that the Society was in support of the new treatment protocol. I'll leave it at that.

Frequency of injections

As I have said, inadequate treatment is by far the biggest source of complaint by members of the Pernicious Anaemia Society. Within that, it is the frequency of replacement therapy injections that concerns members most, and it is in this area that the difference between scientific evidence and patient experience becomes most obvious. While some doctors are prepared to listen to their patients and prescribe more frequent injections than is usual, most GPs will refuse to depart from the guidelines for treatment as set out in the *BNF* and this, in turn, leads to inequality of treatment, strained relationships between doctors and patients, and unnecessary suffering. It's a constant source of frustration for the Pernicious Anaemia Society, which has to deal with this problem on a daily basis.

The USA's Centers for Disease Control and Prevention has this to say about the different types of injections and their frequency:

> Few side effects have been reported, and patient acceptance is generally high. Anecdotally, the subcutaneous route causes less burning than does the intramuscular route (Carmel RA, New York Methodist Hospital [personal communication] 2006–2007). Regimens for parenteral

administration vary. An approach suggested by Stabler and Allen is 1 milligram (1000 mcg) weekly for eight weeks, then once monthly for life.[6]

Monthly injections that are prescribed in the United States are of cyanocobalamin. In the UK, hydroxocobalamin is used which is supposed to be retained in the body for longer, though I have not been able to find any evidence of this. (This doesn't mean it doesn't exist; it's just that I have not been able to find anything other than vague statements relating to treating pregnant women.) Similarly, it is stated that intramuscular injections are retained for longer than the much less painful, and easily self-administered subcutaneous injections.

To fully understand this strange situation of different treatment protocols it is necessary to establish some basic facts about the symptoms of pernicious anaemia.

Michael and Jenna's stories

There's something not fully appreciated by medical practitioners that may be an indicator why the frequency of replacement therapy is such an issue. I'd like to introduce you to Michael. Michael was 45 years old when he visited his doctor about a condition quite unrelated to pernicious anaemia. His doctor asked for a full blood count and a few days after giving blood Michael received a telephone call from the health centre asking him to make an appointment to see his doctor. A day or so later Michael was sitting in front of his GP who seemed very concerned.

'How much alcohol do you consume?' asked the doctor.

'Oh, I usually go to the pub on Sunday afternoons after playing football,' was his reply. The doctor frowned.

'How much do you consume during the week?'

'Hardly anything – it's usually only on a Sunday lunchtime. Why, is there something wrong?'

'Your red blood cells are incredibly enlarged,' said the doctor, 'which indicates alcohol abuse – are you sure you don't consume large amounts?'

'I only have two or three pints of beer on a Sunday,' repeated Michael.

The interrogation continued.

'Do you feel unusually tired?'

'No.'

'Do you ever get short of breath?'

'No – not at all.'

The doctor looked at Michael who appeared fit and healthy.

'I want to run another blood test to check your vitamin B_{12} levels – make an appointment with the nurse.'

The day after having a sample of blood taken Michael received a telephone call on his mobile. He was told that his vitamin B_{12} levels were virtually non-existent, that he had pernicious anaemia and that he must make an immediate appointment with the practice nurse to start receiving B$_{12}$ injections. Michael had none of the symptoms yet his B$_{12}$ levels were rock bottom. I asked Michael how often he received his injections.

'It's supposed to be every three months but often I forget and it goes to four, even five months,' he told me.

Contrast Michael's story with Jenna who self-injects three times a day as recommended by her physician, whom she paid to see.

'I inject 1 ml of 5 mg/ml methylcobalamin three times a day. It stops me from having suicidal thoughts,' she told me. Jenna is a practising GP.

Many members of the Pernicious Anaemia Society regularly self-inject using subcutaneous injections rather than the more uncomfortable intramuscular injections usually given by the nurse. Here's what the survey found:

Of those individuals receiving B$_{12}$ by injection, <1% were being treated more than once a day; 1% were being treated daily; 2% weekly; 9% monthly; 15% twice-monthly; 50% once every 3 months; and 10% were being treated at some 'other' frequency.

Don't forget that these figures only apply to patients living in the UK, where the recommended treatment set out in the *BNF* is 1 mg of hydroxocobalamin every three months unless there is any neurological involvement, in which case the injection should be given every two months (and initially every other day until symptoms no longer improve – see above). And while we are talking of the *BNF*, take a look at this email that I received in the run-up to a Parliamentary reception that we held in February 2015.

Email from a consultant physician

I am interested in your campaign to raise awareness of the need of some PA patients for cobalamin dosage more frequently than every three months. I am myself a consultant physician, now retired, and I was diagnosed with PA (classic autoimmune PA with IF antibodies) over 20 years ago when I was 50. When I was diagnosed one of the first things I did was to ring a general practitioner friend who I knew had suffered from PA for several years. Straight away he said to me, 'Don't take any notice of the *BNF* guidance that B_{12} should be given every three months.' He said he took his every month, and if he forgot a dose, his family would notice he was getting miserable and would say, 'Dad, have you had your injection lately?' (Sadly, my friend has since died of an unrelated condition.)

It turned out that I found I just could not last three months between injections as my symptoms always returned between four and eight weeks after my dose. In my case I notice a sore mouth, especially my tongue, a peppery taste, and mouth ulcers, and these disappear within 48 hours of a dose of B_{12}. I now don't wait for the symptoms to appear, and just give myself an injection on the first of every new month. My GP only once queried the frequency with which I was using the cobalamin, and I managed to persuade him to let me carry on without having further investigation by a haematologist as to whether it was necessary, which I knew would be unhelpful.

Have you enquired about practice in other countries with regard to frequency of B_{12} injections? Anecdotally, I recall once or twice asking doctors who worked with me but who

---

> had been trained overseas about this topic, and finding they were surprised that in Britain doctors were giving B$_{12}$ so infrequently.
>
> Keep up your excellent work.

The email addresses two issues. Firstly, different countries have different treatment regimens – for instance, in the USA 1 mg of cyanocobalamin is prescribed every month whereas in the UK hydroxocobalamin is prescribed every three months; because hydroxocobalamin is supposedly retained by the body longer than cyanocobalamin, though I haven't been able to find any evidence of this. Secondly, it is often not the patient who notices a return of the symptoms of B$_{12}$ deficiency but the patient's family, friends or work colleagues. And this is important because unfortunately, when patients return to their doctor to ask for another injection before their next one is scheduled, they are routinely offered anti-depressants – I know this because of the great many instances where members of the Society have told me of their experiences.

We also know that the *BNF* used to recommend that 1 mg of hydroxocobalamin be administered every month, but this was changed to every two months in 1974 and then to every three months in 1984. I recently met with the Director of the *BNF* and asked her if we could please revert to pre-1974 guidelines. The answer was an emphatic 'no', because the decision to change the regimen from every month to every two months and then to every three months would have been based on 'hard scientific evidence'. And of course some patients, like Michael, manage perfectly well on the existing recommended treatment. The Director of the *BNF* also pointed out to me that some doctors would prefer the treatment to be changed to every six months or even a year.

Cyanocobalamin versus hydroxocobalamin

The merits and demerits of different types of B_{12} injection have been debated and discussed by various online forums over the years and it seems clear that some patients respond better to treatment with one particular form of B_{12} injection than others. Some patients in the UK find that their symptoms are alleviated to a greater degree when they use cyanocobalamin rather than hydroxocobalamin, which is what is usually prescribed in the UK. Meanwhile, there are members of the Pernicious Anaemias Society living in mainland Europe who respond better to hydroxocobalamin. It is easy to attribute this to some sort of perceived benefit from one type of B_{12} than another and if there were just a handful of isolated cases this could be considered as an explanation. However, the sheer number of patients who prefer one type of B_{12} to others means that again there is a need for this to be fully investigated. There is a danger that patients being supplied with B_{12} from countries other than their own may experience different outcomes. Here's what one group of researchers has to say about this:

> Different vitamin B_{12} drugs may result in different treatment outcomes, and caution should be taken when treating patients with vitamin B_{12} drugs from other countries.[7]

One thing is clear: both cyanocobalamin and hydroxocobalamin require adequate amounts of folate to be present to convert either of the forms of B_{12} to methylcobalamin. And it is methylcobalamin that is the preferred type of B_{12} injection where it is available.

Allergic reactions to injections

While on the subject of injections it is important to include the vexed issue of allergies. The most common allergic reaction to injections of B_{12} is a slight rash, though this can be more severe in some patients.

Other side effects include strong-smelling urine, diarrhoea, heart palpitations and itchy skin. Thankfully, severe allergic reactions to the injections are rare but they do occur and can lead to anaphylactic shock – which is why you should never self-inject any type of B$_{12}$ for the first time on your own. Ideally, your first injection should be delivered by a doctor or other medical professional who will be able to deal with any adverse reaction. At the very least, any injection being self-administered for the first time should be done under the supervision of a medical professional. I know of one member of the Pernicious Anaemia Society who had a reaction of this sort when she received her first injection from her health centre nurse; it led to her being admitted to hospital and she visited the Society's office to tell me of her ordeal. It may be that a patient is allergic to a particular type of B$_{12}$ he or she receives. Some patients can tolerate cyanocobalamin but not hydroxocobalamin[8] and so changing the type of B$_{12}$ given might have the desired effect – but remember, methylcobalamin is not licensed for use in the UK.

If the patient is unable to tolerate either of the usually prescribed injections then the only way forward is for him or her to undergo a desensitisation process which involves receiving very small doses of diluted B$_{12}$ (either as hydroxocobalamin or cyanocobalamin), initially every 15 minutes but becoming less frequent as the days progress, whilst at the same time the doses become more concentrated. One desensitising programme involving two patients with pernicious anaemia took place over 49 days.[9]

Although the method described above is a possibility, unfortunately there is no established protocol for desensitising patients to available forms of B$_{12}$ and the patient and physician will have to find some alternative treatment:

> Due to the small number of cases in the literature there is no standard treatment regimen or desensitisation procedure for the vitamin B12 allergy yet. Therefore, we suggest that our

case report may contribute to the formation of standardised desensitisation protocol in vitamin B12 allergy.[10]

Like many other aspects of pernicious anaemia, this is one more area where more research needs to be conducted.

Alternative delivery methods

Where patients are unable to convince their doctor that they need a more individually tailored treatment programme but are reluctant to self-inject for whatever reasons, they often turn to alternative delivery methods to supplement their injections. Demand for these products means that there is now a wide variety of alternative ways for ensuring that patients have adequate levels of B_{12} in their body. And whilst there has been some, perhaps inadequate, research into the efficacy of large oral doses of B_{12}, none of the other products that have been produced have had their efficacy assessed. These products acknowledge the fact that patients with pernicious anaemia are unable to absorb B_{12} in their digestive tract and so concentrate on alternative routes into their bloodstream.

Sub-lingual etc

Sub-lingual products are administered under the tongue where the vitamin crosses a thin membrane that is found there and enters the bloodstream. These sub-lingual products include lozenges and sprays. Other methods developed on the same basis include nasal sprays, nasal drops, skin patches, anal suppositories, intra-urethral suppositories and drops, intravaginal pessaries, and even underarm drops or powders.[11]

Sub-lingual sprays can be useful supplements to more traditional treatments. Usually I suggest that patients buy the potent B_{12} Boost sub-lingual spray that is available at high street stores in the UK, then take the spray with them when they next visit their doctor and discuss with him or her using the spray to supplement between injections. It is important that the patient discusses this with his or her doctor because using the spray will mean that any future test to assess his or her B$_{12}$ status will, or at least should, show a high or extremely high level of B$_{12}$ in his/her blood. Some doctors are perfectly happy with their patients supplementing like this though they would not allow more frequent injections. I'll leave you to ponder on why this is so.

As well as meeting with the editors of the *BNF* in November 2014, I also met with representatives of the UK's Medicines and Healthcare Products Regulatory Agency (MHRA) and asked if they could help patients get treatment according to their individual need. However, I was told that while the agency approved new medicines they were not involved in developing new treatments themselves. And when you take into consideration the immense costs involved in bringing a new treatment, such as methylcobalamin, to market, and the very poor financial gain for pharmaceuticals from this as yet unlicensed form of B$_{12}$, it is little wonder that there is no interest from pharmaceutical companies to develop new treatments. This is why alternative delivery methods, such as nasal sprays or sub-lingual sprays, are not available from GP surgeries, at least not in the UK.

Powder

Another way in which methylcobalamin is supplied to patients is in powder form which the user rehydrates using sterile water and then injects (or gets a friend or relative to) using a sub-cutaneous injection. Obviously the user will need to ensure that the powder is from a reliable source and of pharmaceutical grade.

Intravenous infusions

This procedure has become a popular treatment. Though it is not provided by the NHS in the UK, it is offered by various doctors and clinics in the private sector. Intravenous vitamin infusions are usually a mixture of vitamin C, B vitamins, magnesium and calcium. They are sometimes referred to as a 'Myers cocktail' after the Baltimore physician who developed the formula in the 1980s. These infusions have made the news lately because a number of 'celebrities' are advocates and some post pictures of themselves receiving a bag full of vitamins that is injected straight into the bloodstream via an intravenous 'drip'. Patients with vitamin B_{12} deficiency have the cocktail of vitamins 'customised' so that they will receive a high dose, and it will be a high dose, of vitamin B_{12} (methylcobalamin). The idea is that the body becomes saturated with the vitamin and patients who have pernicious anaemia can then self-inject themselves regularly to keep themselves 'topped up'. This is what I do – I had an initial infusion that was administered by a doctor – a consultant anaesthetist, actually – and was then provided with a 30 ml bottle of 5 mg/ml methylcobalamin. I now inject 1 ml twice a week using a small insulin needle. Immediately after the infusion I was told to inject three times a day. This approach to treatment is used by several medical professionals who are members of the Pernicious Anaemia Society.

There are many anecdotal examples of patients feeling enormous benefits from the infusions, including myself. I remember that by the time I returned home from having my infusion I could feel my trousers rubbing against my legs and the pedals in my car under my feet for the first time in seven years, and although I still get very tired in the afternoons, the awful 'fog days' that I used to have to endure are a thing of the past. However, anecdotes are not evidence and, like most things to do with pernicious anaemia, this increasingly popular form of treatment needs to be investigated thoroughly.

The method itself is receiving a good deal of attention – at the time of writing:

> There are currently 274 clinical research trials employing intravenous micronutrient therapy. About half of these concern treatment or prevention of cancer. The remainder cover a wide range of medical and health conditions.[12]

There is a growing number of clinics that offer B$_{12}$ infusions, and that growing number can be seen to be the market responding to an increase in demand. However, even though the number of clinics and practitioners is growing, demand still outstrips supply, which means that the procedure is costly (between £200 and £600) depending on the time taken up with a consultation, tests etc., and there is often a waiting list of between a few weeks and a few months. You should always ensure that the practitioner is a qualified and registered doctor as I am aware that some 'clinics' are offered by hairdressers and beauty therapists. What would they do if the patient suffered a severe allergic reaction?

With the exception of oral tablets, all of the methods outlined above promise to be viable methods of treatment for patients with pernicious anaemia because they bypass the stomach. And yet the efficacy of these novel delivery methods has not been subjected to any thorough evaluation, and any evaluation would not be as straightforward as it might first seem.

Efficacy of treatments

The problem in evaluating the efficacy of treatments – including injections – goes back to the fact that some patients have high levels of B$_{12}$ yet are still symptomatic while others have low, or even very low, serum B$_{12}$ levels and yet have none of the symptoms. Some patients feel better using particular forms of B$_{12}$ than others and some need much more frequent supplementation than others.

A paper published in 1992 described how a female patient who had undergone a full gastrectomy – her stomach had been removed – developed not only megaloblastic anaemia but also urinary and faecal incontinence and peripheral neuropathy in her arms and legs. The doctors used intramuscular B_{12} that improved her blood picture but didn't cure the incontinence or neuropathy. The doctors changed their tactics and started to use intravenous B_{12} injections with quite remarkable outcomes:

> While the haematological abnormalities were improved by administration of a total dose of 17 mg of intramuscular mecobalamin,[vi] the neurological abnormalities remained unchanged. Five months later, a total dose of 7.5 mg of mecobalamin was injected intravenously over a period of five weeks, although the serum level of vitamin B_{12} was greater than 1180 pmol/l. Immediately after initiation of the therapy, the urinary and faecal incontinence were gradually improved, and were completely cured within two months. The peripheral neuropathy was also ameliorated. The effectiveness of intravenous vitamin B_{12} injection for the neurological abnormalities due to vitamin B_{12} deficiency is emphasized.[13]

Both methods of addressing the lack of B_{12} were successful in rectifying the patient's anaemia but only the intravenous method of delivery addressed the problem of incontinence and neuropathy, though there is no explanation for this.

Any evaluation of the efficacy of the treatment method would therefore need to be based on the response of the patient overall and not just on his or her blood picture. There are a number of theories

---

[vi] This is another term for methylcobalamin.

surrounding this, with some doctors believing that regardless of the level of B$_{12}$ in the patient's serum, he or she might not be responding to treatment because of ineffective or inadequate transcobalamin receptors on cells. I don't want to go into this area any deeper because I don't understand it, but I know that this is the explanation given by some doctors when they are told that some patients are still symptomatic with high levels of serum B$_{12}$ and need more frequent treatment than is usually given. There's certainly something more going on than simply rectifying the patient's abnormal blood picture.

IMPORTANT – You should *always* discuss with your doctor any alternative treatment that you are considering before commencing with it.

The placebo effect

Research into the efficacy of treatments is complicated by alleged 'placebo' effects. A placebo is an imagined benefit from taking a medicine that is, in fact, ineffective. When patients ask their doctor for more frequent injections they are usually told that they don't need more than has been prescribed and that they (the patients) are 'imagining' that they need more. Why should doctors think that a patient is imagining that more frequent injections benefit them?

The reason is quite simple to understand if you think back to how the patient would have been diagnosed with pernicious anaemia in the first place. He or she would have been found to have a low level of serum B$_{12}$ (though we now know that there is controversy over what constitutes a low level), and as a result would have had abnormally large red blood cells (perhaps) and consequently would also have had low amounts of haemoglobin in his/her blood; as a result the patient would (probably) have had the symptoms of B$_{12}$ deficiency. Now, once the patient had begun to receive replacement therapy injections, his or her serum B$_{12}$ levels would have increased markedly and, as far as doctors were concerned, providing that he/she also had adequate levels of iron and folate, his/her blood would have returned to normal. This sequence of events is especially true of haematologists who will have witnessed all of the indicators of a deficiency of B_{12} caused by pernicious anaemia disappearing. This will lead them to believe that either the patient is 'imagining' that they still have the symptoms, or that they have some other disease.

From there it is only a short hop to the doctor deciding that the patient is experiencing a 'placebo effect' from more frequent injections. Of all the responses made by doctors to requests for more frequent replacement therapy injections, this 'placebo effect' is the one that annoys me most. Doctors put their faith in scientific evidence to arrive at a diagnosis and yet they are all too eager to attribute the patient benefiting from more frequent injections to a placebo effect when there is no scientific foundation for telling the patient that his or her symptoms are imaginary.

I'm not blaming doctors for their reaction because, after all, the patient's blood will have been examined by a laboratory and shown to be 'normal', but it would be helpful, and interesting, to find out if patients are indeed imagining that they need more frequent injections. And remember, it is often not the patient who notices his or her symptoms reappearing but those who live or work with him/her.

Just before Christmas 2014 I met with a senior and much respected figure in the world of haematology. I mentioned that the biggest cause of complaint among members of the Pernicious Anaemia Society was not being treated by their doctor according to their individual needs. I was given an immediate response that it was because 'they must be suffering from another disease' and that 'something else was the cause of their symptoms because their blood would have returned to normal.' The speaker didn't actually think about what I said or ponder why it could be so – rather he simply dismissed any need for anything other than a standard treatment.

And, as he's a haematologist (a blood specialist, not a general physician or a neurologist), I can understand his reaction.

This leads us on to another interesting, though for some doctors inconvenient, aspect of the treatment of pernicious anaemia – often, even though the patient is receiving more than enough replacement B_{12}, he or she will *still* experience the worst effects of the symptoms of the disease even though his/her blood picture will show nothing untoward. There seem to be a number of reasons why this is so; we will look at these next.

Post-treatment symptoms

The logical treatment for pernicious anaemia is to provide the patient with an 'external' source of B_{12} as he or she will not be able to absorb the vitamin from food. It is again logical to assume that, once the patient's B_{12} levels have returned to normal and that there is no deficiency in anything else, that the symptoms of pernicious anaemia will recede altogether. Yet this is not always the case. I still experience the symptoms of the disease, though not as severely as when I was eventually diagnosed, while some patients make a remarkably full recovery and never see a return of their original symptoms in any shape or form. So why is it that some patients do not make a full recovery and continue to suffer the worst effects of vitamin B_{12} deficiency? It seems there could be a number of causes, though there is no general agreement. The first of these involves some complex biochemistry and mutant genes.

Methylenetetrahydrofolate reductase (MTHFR)

I have to confess that, despite the best efforts of a variety of very clever scientists, I still don't fully understand the complex chemistry here but, suffice it to say, this enzyme plays an important part in the *methylation* process which leads to the production of the active forms of B_{12}. I'll do my best to make this simple.

The main form of folate in the body is 5-methyltetrahydrofolate (5MTHF), which is the biologically active folate used at the cellular level for the methionine cycle and the regulation of homocysteine. High levels of homocysteine are linked with increased risk of heart attack, stroke and dementia and are a good indicator of low B_{12} status. 5,10-Methylenetetrahydrofolate (5,10MTHF) is an important intermediate form that is required for DNA repair and DNA and RNA synthesis. There is a specific enzyme that carries out the conversion of 5,10-MTHF to 5-MTHF and it's called – wait for it – methylenetetrahydrofolate reductase (MTHFR).

Depending on geographical location around 16% of people will have a faulty gene associated with MTHFR which *could* lead to problems with the patient's ability to process this conversion, meaning that they won't be able to regulate homocysteine production efficiently, with all the consequences that comes with it. This theory is at the cutting edge of biochemistry and medicine and whilst some doctors have made the study of MTHFR their life's work, there is a need for this issue to be explored further.

It is worth noting here that some doctors are vehemently opposed to supplementing with folic acid because it also needs to undergo this conversion into 5-MTHF, and if this doesn't happen the patient will be putting him or herself at risk of having elevated homocysteine. An internet search will yield much more information about this but don't expect it to be easily understood unless you have some scientific knowledge, which I lack. However, if all of this has led to you discovering the hidden biochemist inside yourself, then here's a diagram (figure 5.1) that might make things clearer – note I say 'might'.

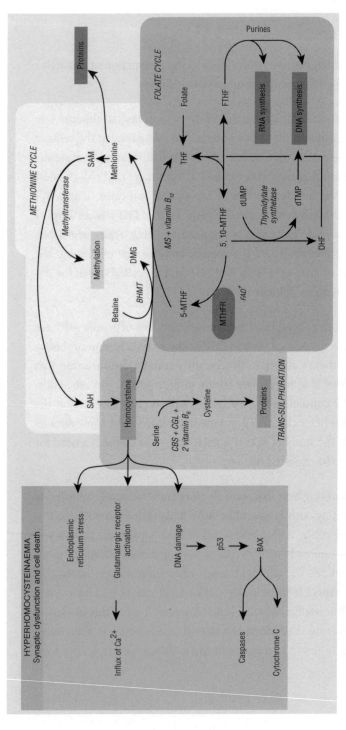

Figure 5.1 MTHFR metabolism: folate cycle, methionine cycle, trans-sulphuration and hyperhomocysteinaemia (Key to abbreviations: 5-MTHFR = 5-methyltetrahydrofolate; 5,10-MTHF = 5,10-methylenetetrahydrofolate; BAX = Bcl-2-associated X protein; BHMT = betaine-homocysteine S-methltransferase; CBS = cystathionine beta synthase; CGL = cystathionine gamma lyase; DHF = dihydrofolate (vitamin B9); DMG = dimethylglycine; dTMP = thymidine monophosphate; dUMP = deoxyuridine monophosphate; FAD = flavine adenine dinucleotide; FTHF = 10-formyltetrahydrofolate; MS = methionine synthase; MTHRF = methylenetetra-hydrofolate reductase; SAH = S-adenosyl-L-homocysteine; SAM = S-adenosyl-L-methionine; THF = tetrahydrofolate)

Brain lesions

I remember talking to a haematologist at an event in London that was all about blood transfusions. When I told him that many patients with pernicious anaemia were still symptomatic even after replacement therapy injections of B_{12} were started he was genuinely startled. He told me that if patients were still symptomatic after their treatment had begun then it was probably due to brain lesions.

Lesions are areas of tissue that have been damaged in some way, so brain lesions are areas of the brain that have been damaged, and one of the causes of brain lesions is autoimmune activity, though I have not been able to identify any source that specifically mentions pernicious anaemia as being a cause. (This is not to say that pernicious anaemia wouldn't cause any brain lesions but rather that this hasn't been fully examined. That haematologist in London probably made the link.) The symptoms of brain lesions are similar to those often familiar to patients with pernicious anaemia and include 'changes in mood, personality, behaviour, mental ability and concentration, along with memory loss or confusion'.[14]

Tailoring treatment to individuals

In the UK the standard treatment for patients with pernicious anaemia is 1 mg/ml intramuscular injection every three months. As we saw earlier in this chapter, the *British National Formulary* (*BNF*) used to state that patients with pernicious anaemia should be given this treatment once a month, but in 1974 this changed to every two months, and then to every three months in 1984. When I met with the Director of the *BNF* in November 2014 I asked if we could revert back to monthly injections. You may remember that she replied that the changes were based on new scientific evidence. She also said that if I could provide her with anything better than anecdotal evidence as to why the injections should be given more frequently, that evidence would be considered by a panel of experts. And that's the root of the problem with this issue – there simply isn't any hard scientific evidence that some patients need more frequent injections than others. I can provide the *BNF* with anecdotal evidence by the bucketful; what I can't do is offer them any hard evidence based on science-based investigations. However, as I write this in late April 2015 we are about to embark on such an investigation with a leading gastroenterologist and his team to see if we can unearth what is going on.

I've just taken a telephone call from a member of the Pernicious Anaemia Society who has told me that she was unable to manage on the three-monthly injection routine and has to inject herself every week because, if she doesn't, the numbness she experiences in her feet and the pins and needles in her hands return. It was ironic that she should telephone just as I had finished typing the heading for this section. This is just one story of the thousands that I am aware of where the patient needs more frequent injections than others in order to be symptom-free. Just why this is so has never been fully investigated but there is an urgent need for this to take place in order to bring an end to unnecessary suffering. Furthermore, that investigation needs to be carried out by somebody who not only knows what they are doing (in that they are medically trained), but also that person needs to have an open mind and be prepared to listen to patients and their families and friends.

There has been some progress and I know that more and more patients are finding that their GP is now adopting a more flexible approach to their treatment. However, for far too many patients with pernicious anaemia this still remains a contentious issue that often leads to a breakdown in the doctor/patient relationship and means patients bypass their physician and find alternative sources of their treatment, often at considerable cost. Still, there is hope that as long as the Pernicious Anaemia Society keeps pushing this issue onto researchers' agendas, something will be done: here's what one GP wrote recently:

> Finally, many clinicians and patients are aware of considerable individual variability in the response to treatment with vitamin B_{12}. Patients often continue to experience mild neurological symptoms, such as poor memory, impaired concentration and fatigue, even after adequate B_{12} replacement. The reason for this is currently unknown, but future research into the interplay between polymorphisms in transcobalamin and its cell membrane receptor might offer some explanation for this curious phenomenon.[15]

Summary

The usually prescribed one-size-fits-all treatment for patients with pernicious anaemia is perfectly suited to some patients but not to others. Some patients need more frequent doses than others and some respond better to different delivery methods and types of B_{12} than others. While patients are quite rightly angry and confused as to why they may have had to wait a long time for a correct diagnosis, they are willing to forgive their physicians in the belief that they will at last get treated, and this will bring an end to their symptoms. They are not so forgiving when they realise that in some cases, though not all, their treatment is inadequate, leaving them frustrated, angry and confused at the thoughtlessness of their physician. The Pernicious Anaemia Society has a policy that states that patients should be given a choice of treatment in terms of delivery method and frequency that is based on their individual need. Hopefully this chapter will go some way to raising awareness of this important issue.

References

1. Centers for Disease Control & Prevention. Natural history and prevalence of vitamin B$_{12}$ deficiency: http://www.cdc.gov/ncbddd/b12/history.html (Accessed 16 March 2015).

2. Van der Voet H, de Boer WJ, Souverein OW, Doets EL, van't Veer P. A statistical method to base nutrient recommendations on meta-analysis of intake and health-related status biomarkers. PLoS ONE 2014; 9(3). doi:10.1371/journal.pone.0093171.

3. Ibid.

4. Darby, WJ, Bridgeforth EB, Le Brocquy J, Clark SL Jr, De Oliveira JD, Kevany J, McGanity WJ, Perez C. Vitamin B$_{12}$ requirement of adult man. *American Journal of Medicine* 1958; 25(5):726–732.

5. Vidal-Alaball J, Butler CC, Cannings-John R, Goringe A, Hood K, McCaddon A, McDowell I, Papaioannou, A. Oral vitamin B$_{12}$ versus intramuscular vitamin B$_{12}$ for vitamin B$_{12}$ deficiency. Cochrane Database Systematic Review 2005. doi:10.1002/14651858. CD004655.pub2, (Accessed 20 April 2015).

6. Centers for Disease Control and Prevention. Managing patients with evidence of a vitamin B$_{12}$ deficiency. http://www.cdc.gov/ncbddd/b12/patients.html (Accessed 20 April 2015).

7. Arendt J, Nexø E. Treatment response in vitamin B$_{12}$ deficiency depends on the chosen vitamin B$_{12}$ preparation. *Ugeskr Laeger* 2011; 173(42):2634.

8. Heyworth-Smith D, Hogan PG. Allergy to hydroxycobalamin, with tolerance of cyanocobalamin. *Medical Journal of Australia* 2002; 177:162.

9. Caballero MR, Lukawska J, Lee TH, Dugué P. Allergy to vitamin B$_{12}$: two cases of successful desensitization with cyanocobalamin. *Allergy* 2007; 62(11):1341–1342.

10. Kartal O, Gulec M, Demirel F, Yesillik S, Caliskaner Z, Sener O. Vitamin B$_{12}$ allergy and successful desensitisation with cyanocobalamin, a case report. *Allergologia et Immunopathologia* 2012; 40(05):324-325.

11. Stoll Foundation. Alternative ways of administering high dose vitamin B_{12}. http://askwaltstollmd.com/phorum/read.php?3,19454 (Accessed 29 March 2015).

12. MedPage Today. Intravenous vitamin therapy: the latest celebrity health fad. http://www.medpagetoday.com/CelebrityDiagnosis/41227 (Accessed 31 March 2015).

13. Kurabayashi H, Kubota K, Kawada E, Tamura K, Tamura J, Shirakura T. Complete cure of urinary and faecal incontinence after intravenous vitamin B_{12} therapy in a patient with post-gastrectomy megaloblastic anaemia. *Journal of Internal Medicine* 1992; 231(3):313–315.

14. WebMD. Brain lesions: causes, symptoms, treatments. http://www.webmd.com/brain/brain-lesions-causes-symptoms-treatments (Accessed 29 March 2015).

15. McCaddon A. Vitamin B_{12} in neurology and ageing; clinical and genetic aspects. *Biochimie* 2013; 95(5):1066-1076.

Chapter 6

Pernicious anaemia, cancer, neurology and psychiatry

Chapter 4 touched on the range of conditions that can exist alongside pernicious anaemia and the possible mis-diagnoses that can occur when patients' symptoms are investigated. This chapter looks in more depth at some of those conditions – stomach cancer and neurological/psychiatric conditions – and their possible relationship to pernicious anaemia.

Stomach cancer

After 'frequency of injections' and 'injections being stopped altogether' the third most common topic of telephone enquiries to the Pernicious Anaemia Society office is a subject that causes panic, anxiety and alarm – the likelihood of patients with pernicious anaemia developing stomach cancer (also known as gastric cancer).

Before we go any further, let's remind ourselves of the role of the stomach in the digestive process. It is in the stomach that the parietal cells produce intrinsic factor and hydrochloric acid and where the chewed-up food you have eaten – the 'bolus' – is changed into 'chyme' before sending it to the small intestine. That acid is powerful and is prevented from burning a hole in the stomach wall by a membrane that coats the wall and the judicious production of bicarbonate. Stomach cancer is different from colon cancer or, as it is sometimes called, bowel cancer, as it occurs at an earlier stage in the digestive tract.

There is a link between pernicious anaemia and stomach cancer and it is an association that has been known for many years. However, there do not seem to be any reliable statistics that prove the likelihood of patients with pernicious anaemia going on to develop stomach cancer. Here's what the United States' Medline Plus website has to say about pernicious anaemia and gastric cancer: 'People with pernicious anemia may have gastric polyps. They are also more likely to develop gastric cancer and gastric carcinoid tumors.' And the website Patient.co.uk confirms this:

> If you have pernicious anaemia, you are about three times more likely to develop stomach cancer than someone without pernicious anaemia. This means that about 4 in 100 people with pernicious anaemia develop stomach cancer (even when the anaemia is treated).

However, Cancer Research UK's website quotes a paper published in 2011[1] that states that: 'Stomach cancer risk is around 7 times higher in people with pernicious anaemia compared with the general population, a meta-analysis showed.'

A meta-analysis is a piece of research that has looked at the results of several studies where the numbers differ. It is a sort of 'averaging out' of the different numerical values. It isn't 100% accurate but it aims to produce a more accurate picture than the individual results. (I know this because I looked it up.) The fact that the authors of the report conducted a meta-analysis is itself an indicator of there being no accurate and reliable data on the likelihood of patients with pernicious anaemia developing stomach cancer.

What is the risk of developing stomach cancer?

So, what is going on? What is the relationship between pernicious anaemia and the chance of patients going on to develop stomach cancer? One doctor who has an interest in the incidences of stomach cancer and pernicious anaemia is Professor Mark Pritchard, a gastroenterologist at Liverpool University. I asked him if he had any reliable figures regarding this.

> It is actually quite difficult to get reliable statistics about this. There are probably a few reasons for this. The first is that the commonest reason for stomach cancer to develop is that a person has been infected for many years with a bug in the stomach called *Helicobacter pylori*. This accounts for many more cases of stomach cancer than pernicious anaemia. However, both *Helicobacter pylori* infection and pernicious anaemia cause the acid-producing parietal cells to disappear from the stomach lining (a condition called atrophic gastritis), and it can sometimes be difficult to distinguish which one has caused this. Thus it is not always possible to say whether a particular case of stomach cancer has arisen as a result of pernicious anaemia.

Then we come back to the problems with the way in which pernicious anaemia is diagnosed and the consequent problems with identifying how many people have 'classic' pernicious anaemia. Mark Pritchard continued:

> The second [reason] is that not everyone who has vitamin B_{12} deficiency has classical autoimmune pernicious anaemia and this can also cause some distortion of the statistics.

So just that one question on the relationship between stomach cancer and pernicious anaemia cannot be easily answered, though Professor Pritchard did go further:

Stomach cancer is not that common in the UK. Approximately 7,500 cases are diagnosed each year and the majority develop as a result of chronic *Helicobacter pylori* infection. Only a very small proportion of the 7,500 people that develop stomach cancer will have pernicious anaemia (actual numbers not known). If the prevalence of pernicious anaemia is 0.1%, this means that there may be 60,000 individuals in the UK who are affected by this condition. Therefore even though there is perhaps a quoted increased risk of 2–3-fold of developing stomach cancer in a patient with pernicious anaemia compared with a normal member of the population, the actual risk of developing stomach cancer in any individual who has pernicious anaemia is very small. This is an example of how an apparently frightening statistic for the population may not have as much of an effect for an individual who has pernicious anaemia.

I think this response is a sensible and level-headed one which gives a reasoned view of the relationship between stomach cancer and pernicious anaemia that will be welcomed by patients who are anxious about this issue.

Stomach neuroendocrine cancer

Professor Pritchard then went on to talk about a different type of stomach cancer:

Another thing that's worth pointing out is that stomach cancer is not the only type of tumour that can develop in patients with pernicious anaemia. A second type of stomach tumour is the neuroendocrine (previously called carcinoid) tumour. This type of tumour is much more common than stomach cancer in patients with pernicious anaemia (maybe affecting 5% or even up to 10% in some series of patients with PA). Moreover, it doesn't develop in patients who have *Helicobacter pylori* infection instead.

It's time to clarify one thing. A 'tumour' is an abnormal growth of tissue – it comes from the Latin 'tumesco' which means to 'swell up'. Another name for a tumour is 'neoplasm' – from the Greek words for 'new' and 'creation', so a tumour is a new growth. Tumour is one of those words that is automatically associated with something bad, which is understandable because one of the four classes of tumours is a malignant or cancerous one. The three other classes of tumour are not cancerous, but benign. Still, with 5–10% of patients with pernicious anaemia standing the chance of developing a neuroendocrine tumour, is it time to worry? Professor Pritchard was reassuring:

> The good news about the stomach neuroendocrine tumours that develop in pernicious anaemia patients is that most of them are small and do not spread from the stomach and most patients do not need specific treatment and can simply be regularly observed. A few patients who have larger tumours may need treatment either by endoscopic or by surgical removal of these polyps to prevent future problems. Unlike stomach cancer, which can be fatal, it is very unusual for someone to die as a result of the gastric neuroendocrine tumours that arise in pernicious anaemia. However, if someone with pernicious anaemia is diagnosed with these tumours I would recommend that they see a doctor who is familiar with treating such patients so that the condition is not over- or under-treated.

Screening for cancer

Now that is good news, but I had another question for Mark Pritchard, and it was this. Given that there is this link between stomach cancer and pernicious anaemia, is there a case for newly diagnosed patients with pernicious anaemia to be automatically investigated for stomach cancer? And secondly, if yes, how could this be done? These were good questions that elicited a detailed response:

> The problem with stomach cancer is that by the time people develop symptoms the tumour is often quite advanced and may not be amenable to surgical removal and thus cure. As pernicious anaemia is thought to increase the risk of someone developing gastric cancer, if a patient who has pernicious anaemia develops symptoms of indigestion it is probably reasonable to suggest that they should have an endoscopy to investigate matters further. Anyone who also has a so-called 'alarm symptom' – namely, vomiting, vomiting of blood, a sensation of food sticking after swallowing (called dysphagia), weight loss or anaemia that is not responding to regular vitamin B$_{12}$ injections – should certainly be referred for an endoscopy.

An endoscopy is the best test for investigating whether a patient has stomach cancer. This involves passing a flexible tube with a camera on the end through the mouth and throat and down the gullet (oesophagus) into the stomach. This allows the endoscopist to see whether there is any problem and also allows him/her to take biopsies to confirm whether any visibly abnormal area in the stomach is cancerous. An endoscopy is relatively quick (it takes on average 10–15 minutes) and can be done either with a local anaesthetic spray to numb the back of the throat or after a small dose of sedation (but it does not usually require a full anaesthetic). You do not need to stay in hospital.

A barium meal is an alternative to an endoscopy, but it is not usually as good a test as it does not allow biopsies to be taken.

If a cancer is diagnosed at endoscopy, additional tests, particularly a CT scan, will usually be required to see whether the cancer has spread from the stomach to other places in the body, such as the liver. This will determine what treatment should be offered.

Because (i) stomach cancer is not that common, (ii) most people with PA don't develop stomach cancer, and (iii) the endoscopy test is sometimes unpleasant and can have risks, current guidelines in the UK do not suggest that everyone who has pernicious anaemia but has no symptoms should have an endoscopy. This is perhaps an area, however, where more research would be helpful.

What we are discussing here is the question of 'screening' patients routinely and it's a topic that patient groups and doctors often differ over. As far as patients are concerned, if a test is available that is able to detect any abnormality early, they would usually want that test performed, even if it is unpleasant. Doctors on the other hand question this routine screening, believing that the results would not justify the financial costs. Of course, there are some routine screening procedures in place – new-born babies are screened for nine rare but potentially dangerous diseases; women are routinely given cervical smears and breast X-rays – but the introduction of more such programmes raises the question of where do you stop? I represent a patient group who run the risk of developing stomach cancer and it's a risk slightly higher than that of the general population, so do I advocate that all patients who have been diagnosed with pernicious anaemia should routinely be offered an endoscopy? Of course I do, and I go further; I believe that patients should undergo the procedure every three years. But I represent a patient group and so the practicalities need not bother me, which is a blessed thing indeed.

Survival rates for cancer

I had one further question to put to Professor Pritchard. If, and I now know that it's a big if, a patient is diagnosed with stomach cancer, what are his or her survival chances? He replied:

> The crucially important point to make is that prognosis is highly dependent on the stage of the tumour at diagnosis. Early tumours are treated with surgery and are potentially curable, whereas tumours which have metastasised (spread) to other organs at the time of diagnosis cannot be surgically removed and the outlook is much poorer.

This is an argument for routine screening of course.

Finally, there's the issue of treating the stomach cancer. Professor Pritchard said:

> I think the main points to make again are that treatment is largely determined by the stage of tumour at diagnosis. If the tumour is confined to the stomach and the patient is fit enough for surgery, that is their best (in fact probably only) chance of cure. Other treatments, such as chemotherapy, are used to treat more advanced tumours, but are unlikely to be curative.

The symptoms of stomach cancer include:

- pain or discomfort in the upper tummy (abdomen), especially after eating
- indigestion (note: most people who have indigestion do not have stomach cancer)
- feeling sick, and being 'off' food
- weight loss and/or loss of appetite
- passing blood out with your stools (faeces).[2]

If you have any or all of the above, it is important that you discuss this with your doctor as soon as possible.

So where does that leave us patients with pernicious anaemia, with regard to the chance of developing stomach cancer? Well, it seems that we do have a slightly increased risk of developing it but it is impossible to give an accurate figure. Certainly, following my discussion with Professor Pritchard, I will not be worrying unduly about developing stomach cancer – but there again, I've only recently undergone an endoscopy which showed everything was fine. As the website of Cancer Research UK puts it: 'Having pernicious anaemia may increase the risk of stomach cancer' and:

> Both pernicious anaemia and familial polyposis are conditions that can run in families. So a few people do inherit conditions which can give them a greater risk of getting stomach cancer in the future.[3]

Note the words 'may' and 'can', which can be applied to almost any disease. The important thing is to be aware of the symptoms and if you experience any, don't ignore them but discuss them with your doctor.

Neurological and psychiatric problems

Vitamin B_{12} deficiency causes various neurological and psychiatric problems. Psychiatric problems range from cognitive and behavioural disturbances to psychosis and dementia. Neurological problems include:

- myelopathy (problems with the spinal cord)
- neuropathy (problems with the patient's nerves)
- weakness
- altered sensory experiences
- loss of balance
- walking difficulties (gait abnormalities).

Psychiatric problems range from cognitive and behavioural disturbances to psychosis and dementia.

The Pernicious Anaemia Society survey found that 'Most individuals (98%) also reported a range of neurological symptoms', including:

- memory loss (78%)
- poor concentration (75%)
- clumsiness (66%)
- pins and needles (66%)
- poor sleep (64%)
- confusion (62%)
- dizziness (59%)
- headaches (52%)
- nominal aphasia (word-finding difficulties) (50%)
- 'shoulder bumps' (frequently bumping into things as a result of balance problems) (48%)
- unable to stand with eyes closed (34%)
- Grierson-Gopalan ('burning feet') syndrome (33%)
- vertigo (33%).

Sub-acute combined degeneration of the cord

Left undiagnosed and untreated, pernicious anaemia can and does lead to severe and irreversible nerve damage. Nerves are composed of electrically responsive cells that transmit electrical and chemical signals to various parts of the body. Nerve cells, or neurons, are composed of three distinct parts – the cell body (soma), dendrites and an axon. We needn't go any further into the field of neurology other than to know that the axon is covered by a fatty substance called myelin. The myelin acts as a sort of insulating covering of the nerve (the 'myelin sheath') and ensures that nerve impulses are transmitted quickly and properly through the body. And in order for the myelin sheath to be both properly formed and remain healthy, vitamin B$_{12}$ is needed. Starved of B$_{12}$ the myelin sheath disintegrates and 'demyelination' takes place – known to doctors as myelopathy. Demyelination is the loss of the myelin sheath insulating the nerves, and is the hallmark of neurodegenerative autoimmune diseases, including, among others, multiple sclerosis.[ii]

The exact mechanism by which the damage to the myelin sheath occurs is not completely understood and we needn't get involved in the debate, but what is known is that one of the consequences of pernicious anaemia going undiagnosed and untreated is that demyelination takes place, which leads in turn to sub-acute combined degeneration (SACD) of the spinal cord secondary to pernicious anaemia.

And there's something else that needs to be understood. If someone is deficient in vitamin B_{12} *and* folate (vitamin B_9), the vitamin B_{12} deficiency must be treated first to avoid precipitating sub-acute combined degeneration of the cord. The reason for this is that giving folic acid first will correct any anaemia but will leave untouched the lack of methylcobalamin, and it is methylcobalamin that is needed for the stability of myelin; correcting anaemia without correcting methylcobalamin deficiency will therefore lead to demyelination and subsequent nerve damage.

The folate trap

The folate trap is a subject of much debate on various social media sites and it involves some complex biochemistry. Someone who knows about the relationship between folate, B_{12} and demyelination is Professor David Smith, Emeritus Professor of Pharmacology at the University of Oxford. I asked Professor Smith to explain just what goes on when a patient's folate deficiency is addressed but not

---

[ii] According to the survey of members of the Pernicious Anaemia Society just under 3% were originally diagnosed as having MS.

his or her B$_{12}$ deficiency, and even though his reply was as simple as possible it is still a little difficult for non-scientists (like me) to understand.

What happens in B$_{12}$ deficiency is that all the folate gets converted into a substance called 5-methyl-tetrahydrofolate (5MTHF), which cannot donate its methyl group to homocysteine because there is insufficient B$_{12}$ to accept the methyl group. So the folate is 'trapped' as 5MTHF and cannot be used either to make methionine – so methylation is inhibited – or to form THF, which is a precursor of RNA and DNA; hence we get megaloblastic anaemia. Giving extra folate will bypass the latter problem and so get rid of the anaemia but will not rescue the methylation. It is the loss of methylation ability that probably causes demyelination, since myelin basic protein needs to be methylated to function properly. So it is the *lack* of methylcobalamin that causes the problem.

And why is this such an issue? Well, if we remember from previous chapters, there's a continuing debate in Europe about the mandatory fortification of flour to prevent neural tube defects. We have already seen that vitamin B$_{12}$ deficiency is a recognised worldwide problem. If people are taking extra folic acid then that could mask not only one of the indicators of B$_{12}$ deficiency that doctors look for – enlarged red blood cells – but also any associated anaemia. And the consequence of that could be that any B$_{12}$ deficiency would go uncorrected, leading ultimately to permanent nerve damage – subacute combined degeneration of the cord secondary to pernicious anaemia.

Again, I'm not saying that fortification of flour with folic acid shouldn't take place; rather what I am trying to get across is that these potentially serious consequences of fortification should be taken into account before any final decision is made.

Consequences

Let's take a look at this serious consequence of pernicious anaemia (and B_{12} deficiency) going undiagnosed and untreated.

- *Sub-acute*[iii] means the condition is between acute (short term) and chronic (long term);
- *Combined* means that both the posterior and lateral columns (of the spinal cord) have undergone deterioration;
- *Secondary* means, in this case, caused by pernicious anaemia.

It's important to realise, however, that it is often not just the spinal cord that is damaged – the brain, peripheral nerves and optic nerves are also prone to mutilation. Patients usually experience a wide range of symptoms and those symptoms can range from mild to severe and can include weak arms and legs, vision changes and tingling and numbness that gets worse the longer the patient is deficient in B_{12}. Pressure, vibration and touch senses are also usually diminished, which is why one of the tests used by doctors to identify any damage to the spinal cord involves running a blunt instrument over the sole of the patient's foot. In a normal healthy person the reaction is that the big toe moves downwards. If the toe reacts by moving upwards, that is a sign of damage to the spinal cord – the Babinski sign. Other symptoms include clumsiness, difficulty thinking and visual disturbances. Involuntary movements, erectile dysfunction and bladder problems are other frequently reported symptoms.

On a positive note, there is some evidence that one particular form of B_{12} – methylcobalamin – does help to repair damage to the nerves.[4] The evidence is rather thin but there is a lot of it and it should be investigated fully.

[iii] Sometimes written without the hyphen as 'subacute'.

Peripheral neuropathy

Peripheral neuropathy occurs when the patient experiences a combination of paraesthesia and numbness in the outer extremities of the body – the ends of arms and legs. Paraesthesia can take the form of pins and needles, tickling and burning sensations. Another less known but often experienced type of paraesthesia is *formication*, which is the feeling that small insects are crawling on or under the skin. (Be careful you don't substitute an 'n' for the fourth letter which could prove embarrassing.)[iv] Peripheral neuropathy also includes the feeling of a limb 'falling asleep' which, when you think of it, is a strange, though common way to describe the loss of sensation in part of, or the whole of, an arm or leg.

Brain shrinkage

Several studies have been conducted into the effect of low B$_{12}$ and the speed at which the brain shrinks leading to diseases such as Alzheimer's and dementia: 'In the present study, we found that an increase in either vitamin B$_{12}$ status or in folate status was associated with a reduced rate of atrophy.'[5] In another study: 'The researchers found that on average the brains of those taking the folic acid, vitamin B$_6$ and B$_{12}$ treatment shrank at a rate of 0.76% a year, while those in the placebo group had a mean brain shrinkage rate of 1.08%.'[6]

It seems to be the case that it is not the high or adequate levels of B$_{12}$ that *directly* slow down the rate of brain atrophy, but rather the lower levels of homocysteine that are a direct result of the adequate or high amount of B$_{12}$ in the patient's blood. Low B$_{12}$ leads to high levels of homocysteine (HCy) which, it is now generally accepted, lead to the patient's brain shrinking: '77/84 cross-sectional studies on >37,000 people showed an association between raised Hcy, or

---

[iv] Formication is derived from the Latin for ant, *formica*.

low-normal B vitamins, and cognitive deficit or dementia'.[7]

As we have discussed before, as doctors become better at keeping people alive, the number of elderly people in the population will increase, and whilst brain shrinkage is a normal result of the ageing process, perhaps it is time to seriously consider introducing a programme of supplementing the elderly with all B vitamins, including B_{12}.

Alzheimer's disease and dementia

There is something important that needs to be understood about these conditions. 'Dementia is a syndrome (a group of related symptoms) associated with an ongoing decline of the brain and its abilities. This includes problems with:

- memory loss
- thinking speed
- mental agility
- language
- understanding
- judgement.'[8]

Alzheimer's disease is the biggest cause of dementia; the other main causes are vascular dementia and dementia with Lewy bodies. Alzheimer Research UK's website lists the symptoms of Alzheimer's disease as:

- regularly forgetting recent events, names and faces
- becoming increasingly repetitive
- regularly misplacing items or putting them in odd places
- confusion about the time of day
- disorientation, especially away from your normal surroundings
- getting lost

- problems finding the right words
- mood or behaviour problems such as apathy, irritability or losing confidence.

If any patient displays some or all of the above then the doctor might diagnose him or her as suffering from Alzheimer's disease *unless* the patient has low serum B_{12}. However, this either/or diagnosis is not universally accepted; one 2003 MD thesis submission said:

> This thesis challenges the assumption that patients with low levels of vitamin B_{12}, or other disturbances of single-carbon metabolism, should be excluded in the diagnosis of AD. These disturbances may well form part of the aetiology of this fascinating but devastating disease.[9]

Surely there should be a thorough investigation into this link between B_{12} and dementia/Alzheimer's disease in order to clarify this confusing situation? One review of this topic concluded that cognition is associated with B_{12} status across much of the normal range, with lower B_{12} levels being associated with poorer cognition and with Alzheimer's disease.[10]

In another trial, people with a diagnosis of 'mild cognitive impairment' were given a range of B vitamins including 0.5 mg of B_{12} daily, for two years; a marked slowing of the rate of brain shrinkage was noted in those parts of the brain that are affected by Alzheimer's disease in the patients given the supplements. Cognitive decline was also slowed. The authors concluded that B_{12} was the key component in the mixture of B vitamins.[11]

Psychosis

It has long been recognised that untreated B_{12} deficiency can and does lead to patients experiencing a wide range of psychiatric manifestations, including all manner of psychotic episodes. 'Psychosis is a mental health problem that causes people to perceive or interpret things differently from those around them. This might involve hallucinations or delusions.'[12]

Hallucinations involve the patient hearing, seeing, feeling, smelling and even tasting things that aren't there. Hearing voices is a common hallucination. Delusions involve the patient believing things that aren't true, such as a neighbour wanting to kill him/her. Whilst much was written in the past about vitamin B_{12} causing psychosis, in recent decades the subject seems to have been largely forgotten and has slipped off the radar of most medical professionals. Indeed, the NHS Choices website lists the following diseases as being known to cause psychotic incidents: HIV and AIDS, malaria, syphilis, Alzheimer's disease, Parkinson's disease, hypoglycaemia, lupus, Lyme disease, multiple sclerosis and brain tumours. There is no mention of pernicious anaemia and B_{12} deficiency, yet it has been widely reported in the past. Here's a selection of quotes from published research papers:

> Earlier surveys have shown that a large number of psychiatric patients have low serum B_{12} levels, ranging from 6-15%.[13]

> In developing countries, underlying B_{12} deficiency should be considered for all patients with new-onset psychosis. As psychosis can precede anaemia and other physical findings, we suggest directly investigating serum B_{12} levels.[14]

> Vitamin B_{12} deficiency, although known to be associated with neuropsychiatric manifestations of varying nature, is an underdiagnosed entity.[15]

However, the authors (Raveendranathan et al, 2013) go on to point out that the serum B_{12} test cannot be relied on to give an accurate picture of a person's B_{12} status:

> The onset of the psychotic symptoms can occur after, in the presence of, or in the absence of, any overt clinical examination findings indicative of vitamin B_{12} deficiency.

And the solution to this is quite simple and was discussed earlier – raise the cut-off point used to define a deficiency in B_{12} :

> The patient described in this report had a relapse of psychotic symptoms while on regular medication with clozapine and improved with parenteral B_{12} supplementation while other medications were unchanged. Psychiatric manifestations in the absence of any overt clinical examination findings indicative of vitamin B_{12} deficiency (including neurological symptoms) are worth noting. Psychiatric manifestations can occur before the levels of vitamin B_{12} are below 175 pg/l, and it has been proposed that the threshold needs to be increased to 550 pg/l.

And there's more:

> A long list of psychiatrically inclined illnesses or symptoms, especially some cases of mood disorder, dementia, paranoid psychoses, violent behaviour and fatigue, have been documented to be caused by vitamin-B_{12} deficiency … these conditions are possibly more commonly caused by B_{12} deficiency than is currently generally accepted, mostly because of a lack of appreciation of the lowest serum-B_{12} level that is necessary to protect against the cerebral manifestations of this deficiency.[16]

> We recommend consideration of B_{12} deficiency and serum B_{12} determinations in all the patients with organic mental disorders, atypical psychiatric symptoms and fluctuation of symptomatology.[17]

I could go on but you should by now be getting the picture. But what of the most common mental health issue encountered by primary care physicians – depression?

Depression

According to the *National Statistics Psychiatric Morbidity Report* of 2001, between 8% and 12% of the population experience depression in any year in the UK which, translated into hard figures, means that between 4.5 and 7 million people will experience depression in some shape or form every year. And that leads me to wonder how many patients diagnosed with depression have B_{12} deficiency as the root cause of their illness? In the early 1990s a group of doctors got together and produced an update on the psychiatric manifestations of B_{12} deficiency.[18] They reviewed a number of studies. They found that:

> Of 53 patients that they saw, five (9%) had psychotic depression and 48 (91%) had major depression alone. In those with psychotic depression, the authors found a statistically significant decrease for B-12 levels, but not for folate.

Another study mentioned in the update concerned 40 patients with cobalamin deficiency. The authors:

> ... found 15 patients who exhibited combinations of the following symptoms: 13 with memory loss; 3 with disorientation; 1 with obtundation [reduced alertness]; 2 with depression; 1 with irritability; 2 with hallucinations; 1 with agitation; 2 with marked personality change; and 1 with abnormal behaviour.

And it isn't only adults who run the risk or psychiatric disorders. The update reported that a team of researchers led by Garewal et al:

studied 23 patients with infantile tremor syndrome. These patients all presented with tremors, pallor, skin pigmentation, regression of milestones, and a subnormal development l quotient. These patients responded to B-12 replacement therapy.

Interestingly, the authors commented:

> regression and persistence of mental retardation in children with infantile tremor syndrome could well be due to a deficient supply of vitamin B-12 to the nervous system during the crucial growing period.

One member of the Pernicious Anaemia Society has witnessed how low B$_{12}$ can lead to psychotic incidents. Here's his story.

Mum's story

In 2002 my mum suffered from peritonitis when her stomach ulcer burst resulting in half of her stomach being surgically removed. As we know now, but she didn't comprehend at the time, the loss of half her stomach would result in her inability to absorb B$_{12}$ naturally.

She was living in an amenity-poor rural cottage on the Algarve in Portugal at the time. It was an idyllic setting for a healthy person; secluded enough to feel cut off from the rest of the world but only a 10 minute drive from the nearest village for supplies. However, for a person suffering from a continued B$_{12}$ deficiency it became a prison fortified by inescapable lunacy.

Fortunately, the day Mum's stomach ulcer burst the weather conditions were conducive to effective telecommunication. The care and treatment were exemplary and she was back on her feet in record time. She was discharged as an in-patient following an in-depth consultation with her surgeon/doctor, none of which she understood directly, and so was translated to her by her 12-year-old son. Then she came straight back to the UK to convalesce with her daughter (my sister).

The initial psychosis could be explained away under the guise of erratic or eccentric behaviour. It began to manifest about nine months after she arrived in England. Her physical equilibrium was disrupted. She would have to hook up with you when walking to avoid staggering from side to side as she made her way from one point to another. She began visiting a well-known local 'fight' pub. This was massively out of character. Mum had never, ever, been a frequenter of public houses, let alone rough ones. She would totter off as soon as the pub opened and start ordering brandies. She would leave the house without telling anyone where she was going which meant my sister would have to go looking for her. After the first frantic search, when she later went missing she was always found in the same place, sipping brandy. On one occasion a member of staff at the pub took my sister to one side and asked how much my mum drank in the morning before attending the pub. When my sister told the staff member that my mum didn't touch a drop of alcohol until she arrived at the pub, the staff member then shared an experience she had had with a relative who was subsequently committed.

Of course, at the time, we all thought that was ridiculous and just put her behaviour down to changing attitude and age.

Mum's behaviour started to become more and more aggressive. She would argue with retail staff and literally took the wheel to ram another car during a parking dispute in a Sainsbury's car park. She also became paranoid. My mum, sister and young nephew visited Ikea and my nephew went to the toilet. Even though my nephew had only been gone a short time, Mum became increasingly vexed and agitated. She became convinced something was 'going on' in the gents and that my nephew was in danger or actually being physically abused. There was absolutely no evidence to support this. After about a minute of pacing (staggering) up and down and banging the wall she ran at the door to the gents to burst in to 'rescue' my nephew, physically pushing two men at the same time.

The psychosis really peaked when she got back to Portugal. By this point she had been without B$_{12}$ for between 12 and 18 months. She started to contact all her grown-up children seeking assistance to sell her home on the Algarve. She went to great lengths to build a case for moving from Portugal to Romania. Her case included property pricing, planned economic growth in the region, generating a sustainable income via renting out part of her property to holiday makers and, as important from a personal perspective, how tired and angry Portugal was making her feel and how difficult she was finding it to live there.

Over time, and as she was becoming more desperate to make the move, the second part of her case was being stressed more than the first. Then came the revelation that she needed blood. She felt weak and ill and put these symptoms down to the stresses of living in Portugal. She remembered that in her youth people with similar conditions were advised by doctors to eat raw liver. Her plan to move, the whole time, had been to go one better and to recruit young staff to work in her property in Romania with a view to imprisoning them and slowly draining them of blood before murdering them and eating their livers.

At this point we all rallied round to see what we had to do. Our youngest brother was present – the one who had translated for Mum when she was discharged from hospital. He took this moment to remember that the doctors had said that she needed to take regular injections of B_{12} following the surgery. In an immediate act of desperation we purchased B_{12} over the counter at the local pharmacist in Portugal and injected her with 20 mg in 2 ml of water for three consecutive days and then weekly thereafter for a month. She returned to 'normal' within three days.

As we saw in Chapter 4, according to the Pernicious Anaemia Society survey, the most frequent original mis-diagnosis of pernicious anaemia was anxiety or depression, with 143 respondents (16%) stating that this is what they were originally told was the reason for their symptoms. This is hardly surprising when you consider the limitations of the test to assess the B_{12} status of the patient, the regrettable way in which some doctors strictly interpret the results and the fact that very few primary care physicians are aware that patients can have pernicious anaemia even if the test for intrinsic factor antibody returns as negative. Doctors will believe that they have exhausted the investigation for pernicious anaemia by running the tests and so find themselves considering the patient to be suffering from a melancholy mood – after all, the blood tests have revealed nothing wrong.

This propensity for doctors to arrive at a diagnosis of depression is reinforced by the symptoms of B$_{12}$ deficiency resembling those of classic depression. Here's how the NHS Choices website explains depression:

> Depression affects people in different ways and can cause a wide variety of symptoms. They range from lasting feelings of sadness and hopelessness, to losing interest in the things you used to enjoy and feeling very tearful. Many people with depression also have symptoms of anxiety.[19]

Patients with undiagnosed pernicious anaemia, and some who have been diagnosed and treated, will relate to those symptoms. They are classic indicators of B$_{12}$ deficiency. According to the survey, 58% of patients reported suffering from mood swings which included feeling low for some period of time. Then there are the physical symptoms of B$_{12}$ deficiency and depression that are remarkably similar:

> There can be physical symptoms too, such as feeling constantly tired, sleeping badly, having no appetite or sex drive, and complaining of various aches and pains.

The severity of the symptoms can vary. At its mildest, you may simply feel persistently low in spirit, while at its most severe, depression can make you feel suicidal and that life is no longer worth living.

In the survey, 22% of respondents admitted to having had suicidal thoughts. It's good to know that this is being investigated. Here's what a paper published in 2005 found:

> Both low folate and low vitamin B$_{12}$ status have been found

in studies of depressive patients, and an association between depression and low levels of the two vitamins is found in studies of the general population. Low plasma or serum folate has also been found in patients with recurrent mood disorders treated by lithium.[20]

And they conclude:

> On the basis of current data, we suggest that oral doses of both folic acid (800 μg daily) and vitamin B_{12} (1 mg daily) should be tried to improve treatment outcome in depression.

Vitamin B_9 and depression

Ah – back to folate. Folate levels also have an impact on mental health:

> Folate deficiency and insufficiency are common among patients with mood disorders and correlate with illness severity. In a study of 2,682 Finnish men, those in the lowest one-third of folate consumption had a 67% increased relative risk of depression. A meta-analysis of 11 studies of 15,315 persons found those who had low folate levels had a significant risk of depression.[21]

And there's also the problem of some people having a faulty gene that means the conversion of 5,10-methylenetetrahydrofolate into 5-methylenetetrahydrofolate, as discussed, in the last chapter, is disrupted:

> Dietary folate must be converted to L-methyl-folate for use in the brain. Patients with a methylenetetrahydrofolate reductase (MTHFR) C677T polymorphism produce a less active form of the enzyme. The TT genotype is associated with major depression and bipolar disorder.[22]

However, it's not only B$_9$ that is associated with depression. A paper from 2010 notes that low B$_{12}$ status can also be a cause of the illness:

> Vitamin B$_{12}$ has been shown to be associated with depression, with higher concentrations of vitamin B$_{12}$ reported to result in better treatment outcomes. Indeed, it has been proposed that vitamin B$_{12}$ has a stronger causal relation to depression than does folate.[23]

Before we leave the subject of depression I want to point out that patients who are suffering from the effects of vitamin B$_{12}$ deficiency, but who remain undiagnosed and treated, will feel depressed. I remember the confusion, sense of hopelessness and despair in the two years it took for me to be eventually diagnosed. Remember that our survey showed that 19% of patients waited five years or more for a diagnosis, so it's little surprise that many of these hapless patients were diagnosed with, and usually offered treatment for, depression. This is just one more compelling reason why there needs to be a thorough review of the way in which pernicious anaemia in particular, and B$_{12}$ deficiency in general, is diagnosed and treated.

Another member of the Pernicious Anaemia Society who has experienced psychiatric problems is Sue, who contacted me and sent me her story when she knew I was preparing this new book. Here it is.

Sue's story

In the summer of 2013 I began feeling dreadfully unwell. I suffered from extreme tiredness, daily headaches, nausea, dizziness and anxiety. I struggled on with everyday life and work but things became more and more difficult as the weeks went by. Then a severe depression took hold of me and after admitting to a close friend that I felt suicidal he insisted that I went to see my NHS GP. The very same day I was admitted to a psychiatric hospital and sectioned under the Mental Health Act. I tried to inform the doctors that I suffered from hypothyroidism and pernicious anaemia and wondered whether one of these was out of sync, but I was not listened to. The only symptoms they paid attention to were the depressive ones. I was wrongly labelled depressed and psychotic but as I lay on my hospital bed I knew that it was all wrong and my body was crying out for something essential to me; I just didn't know what it was at that time. After a week of being in hospital I was given my routine vitamin B_{12} injection and hey presto, within a few hours I felt so much better – alive, energetic, calm and more stable.

The doctors and nurses insinuated that it was too soon, that I couldn't have recovered from my severe depressive episode and they refused to believe that I was well. Unfortunately, my well feelings did not last as I had been denied my thyroid medication and quickly became hypothyroid and very unwell again, and the depressive symptoms returned. I was also given strong mind-altering drugs, an antidepressant and an antipsychotic, which did nothing to alleviate my physical symptoms. I needed my thyroid medication and vitamin B_{12}. After one month in hospital, unbelievably one psychiatrist wanted to have me re-sectioned for up to six months. I could not let this happen; I needed to get home and quickly so that I could work out myself what was going wrong and get well. It took all my strength to let the panel of professionals believe that I was well, that I was not a risk to myself or others and could be allowed home. Thankfully, I was discharged from hospital.

Back at home I still felt dreadful and had mental health

professionals visiting me on a daily basis, none of whom listened to my physical symptoms, just focused on my mental health. After struggling for another two weeks I started to do some research on pernicious anaemia. I read with great interest that the regime of three-monthly injections that I was prescribed by the NHS was not enough for many people. Two days later I self-injected with vitamin B_{12}, hydroxocobalamin. Within two hours, I felt a surge of energy, my headache that I had had for weeks had gone, I felt calm, stable and well. I cleaned my house from top to bottom; I contacted my place of work and returned to work the very next day. I had wasted six weeks of my life; I had been given strong mind-altering medication and had not been listened to by the very professionals who are there to support you. All I needed was a simple vitamin B_{12} injection. It is wrong that this essential medication is denied to so many people and it is unbelievable that many health professionals are not educated on this simple, effective and essential treatment.

Screening for B_{12} deficiency

So, as we have seen, a deficiency in vitamin B_{12} could be the under-lying cause of a patient suffering from a wide range of symptoms that are associated with one of a number of psychiatric illnesses. This raises the question should *all* patients suffering from one or more of the many illnesses that are considered to be psychiatric routinely have their B_{12} status investigated as a matter of course? It's a question that I put to Professor Rob Poole, of Bangor University and Chairman of the Executive Committee of the Royal College of Psychiatrists in Wales. He told me:

There are a number of problems with routinely screening all patients who present with symptoms that could be due to a mental health problem. The first is that we work with a wide range of patients with varying symptoms and it would be difficult to know who would be included in any screening programme. There are a number of other relatively uncommon physical problems that can mimic or exacerbate mental health problems, and it is hard to know which ones merit screening.

Secondly, there is the problem of the enormous cost involved in routinely screening all patients. Thirdly, as you know, there are serious questions about the accuracy of the current assay used to determine B_{12} status in patients – there's simply no guarantee that such a screening programme would be effective in identifying patients who are genuinely B_{12} deficient.

These are, of course, valid points but I pointed out that the costs of screening all patients for B_{12} deficiency would be offset by the costs associated with unnecessary hospitalisation, expensive medicines, consultations etc.

I'm not saying that screening doesn't happen, but at present it is restricted to certain populations or types of problem. For example, when people have symptoms suggestive of dementia, I screen for B_{12} amongst a number of other tests. For the most part, however, we order the tests based on 'clinical suspicion'. This means that when the doctor suspects that some or all of the patient's symptoms might be attributable to a B_{12} deficiency, then a full blood count *and* vitamin B_{12} status would be investigated – not as a matter of course, but when there is a clinical suspicion.

During our discussion it was pointed out to me that, unlike 20 years ago, not all mental health patients will automatically see a psychiatrist; some patients will be assessed and treated by other mental health professionals, such as nurses or nurse practitioners. Professor Poole continued:

> There may be a case for routine screening where the patient isn't referred to a psychiatrist and maybe this would be a worthwhile exercise; and certainly screening programmes are becoming more common in medicine, but such programmes aren't 100% successful and they can, and do, miss patients.

Simply introducing a screening programme that would assess the B$_{12}$ status in all patients and potential patients in the mental health sector was not likely to be a simple and effective as I first thought. I changed tack and asked Professor Poole, in general, how aware psychiatrists and psychiatric nurses are that low B$_{12}$ can and does cause psychosis?

> I honestly don't know – and it would depend on what you mean by psychosis; if you mean major behavioural changes, then I would think that most, if not all, experienced psychiatrists would know that low levels of B$_{12}$ can and do cause behavioural changes, but I don't know how many other mental health professionals would be aware of that fact.

There was a pause before Rob added:

> I'm sure we miss cases – I encountered a patient a few years back whose odd and irrational behaviour was caused by very low levels of B$_{12}$ – and he was picked up even though there was no evidence of macrocytosis whatsoever.

Ah! We were back to the problems with the current B$_{12}$ test – and that led me to my next question, one that was very revealing. I asked Professor Poole whether psychiatrists are aware of the problems with the current B_{12} assay that leads to as many as 35% of patients who have had their B_{12} tested being told their status is fine whereas in reality it is not. His answer was understandably quite vague:

> I don't know for certain, but I don't think they are.

I mentioned the new guidelines from the BCSH that recommend that doctors ignore the B_{12} test result if there is any discordance between the patient's symptoms and the test result. His comment was in line with the response from other medical professionals that I had discussed the new guidelines with:

> Ah, guidelines! The problem is that there are so many guidelines out there, that many only really get read by those with a real interest in that area – maybe that's where your Society could help by raising awareness among medical professionals of the problems faced by your members due to the inaccuracy of the current B_{12} assay.

It was exactly the same point made to me by the Chairman of NICE[v] a few months earlier. I had one final question. I asked if there were any statistics available on the incidence of low B_{12} status among patients undergoing psychiatric treatment? He replied:

> Not that I'm aware of, and if any audit has been carried out then it is unlikely to be very robust.

So there we have it – introducing a screening programme for all patients suspected of having some kind of psychiatric issue is not without problems, and there is a need to raise awareness among mental health professionals of the possibility that a patient's symptoms could be caused by B_{12} deficiency, and that they shouldn't rely on the current test to give an accurate picture of the patient's B_{12} status.

---

[v] National Institute for Health and Care Excellence, UK.

Stephen Maddern is a lifelong friend and, as I am writing, he is nearing retirement after 35 years working in the field of mental health as a psychiatric nurse. I met Steve for the first time in many years recently. I asked him what he and his colleagues knew about vitamin B$_{12}$ deficiency and mental health.

'Not a lot really – it's so rare,' he replied, before adding that in his career he hadn't come across a single case of a patient suffering from one of the many forms of mental illness because of low vitamin B$_{12}$. I pointed out to him that that didn't mean that none of the hundreds, maybe thousands, of patients that had been put in his care hadn't been suffering because of a vitamin deficiency. 'Fair point,' he said.

Summary

Stomach cancer, neuropsychiatric conditions, psychosis and dementia are all causes of concern for patients with pernicious anaemia. Whilst there is some evidence that there is an increased risk of patients with the disease going on to develop stomach cancer, that risk is only marginally above that of the general population and, as Professor Pritchard pointed out, it is thankfully still rare in the UK. Patients are not currently routinely screened for early onset of stomach cancer, but that might change in the future; even today, there is nothing to stop patients from asking their GP to arrange for an endoscopy to be carried out.

There is a compelling case that all psychiatric patients, whether in- or out-patients, should have their B$_{12}$ status checked – preferably with an accurate assay. New developments in the diagnosis and treatment of pernicious anaemia and vitamin B$_{12}$ deficiency are addressed in Chapter 8, but before that we will leave the medical detail aside and look in Chapter 7 at some of the social costs of pernicious anaemia.

References

1 Landgren AM, Landgren O, Gridley G, Dores GM, Linet MS, Morton LM. Autoimmune disease and subsequent risk of developing alimentary tract cancers among 4.5 million US male veterans. *Cancer* 2011; 117:1163–71.

2 NHS Choices. Stomach cancer – symptoms. http://www.nhs.uk/Conditions/Cancer-of-the-stomach/Pages/Symptoms.aspx (Accessed 17 April 2015).

3 Cancer Research UK. Is stomach cancer hereditary? http://www.cancerresearchuk.org/about-cancer/cancers-in-general/cancer-questions/is-stomach-cancer-hereditary (Accessed 15 April 2015).

4 Hooper M. *Pernicious anaemia: the forgotten disease*. London: Hammersmith Books, 2012.

5 Smith DA, Smith SM, de Jager CA, Whitbread P, Johnston C, Agacinski G, Oulhaj A, Bradley M, Jacoby R, Refsum H. Homocysteine-lowering by B vitamins slows the rate of accelerated brain atrophy in mild cognitive impairment: a randomized controlled trial. *PLoS One* 2010; 5(9): e12244. doi:10.1371/journal.pone.0012244

6 Alzheimer's Research UK. B vitamins halve brain shrinkage rate in people with memory impairment. http://www.alzheimersresearchuk.org/b-vitamins-halve-brain-shrinkage-rate-in-people-with-memory-impairment (Accessed 7 April 2015).

7 Smith AD. The worldwide challenge of the dementias: A role for B vitamins and homocysteine? *Food Nutrition Bulletin* 2008; 29: S143-S172.

8 NHS Choices. About dementia. http://www.nhs.uk/conditions/dementia-guide/pages/about-dementia.aspx (Accessed 20 April 2015).

9 McCaddon A. Vitamin B12 deficiency and Alzheimer's disease. MD thesis, University of Sheffield 2003; page 232.

10 Smith AD, Refsum H. Vitamin B-12 and cognition in the elderly. *American Journal of Clinical Nutrition* 2009, 89(suppl.): 707S-711S.

11 Douaud G, Refsum H, de Jager CA, Jacoby R, Nichols TE, Smith SM, Smith AD. Preventing Alzheimer's disease-related gray matter atrophy by B-vitamin treatment. *Proceedings of the National Academy of Science USA* 2013, 110: 9523-9528.

12 NHS Choices. Psychosis. http://www.nhs.uk/conditions/Psychosis/Pages/Introduction.aspx (Accessed 8 April 2015).

13 Rajkumar AP, Jebaraj P. Chronic psychosis associated with vitamin B12 deficiency. *Journal Associated Physicians India* 2008; 56:115–6.

14 Ibid.

15 Raveendranathan D, Shiva L, Venkatasubramanian G, Rao MG, Varambally S, Gangadhar BN. Vitamin B12 deficiency masquerading as clozapine-resistant psychotic symptoms in schizophrenia. *Journal Neuropsychiatry Clinical Neuroscience* 2013; 25:2.

16 Dommisse J. Subtle vitamin-B12 deficiency and psychiatry: a largely unnoticed but devastating relationship? *Medical Hypotheses* 1991; 34(2):131–140.

17 Durand C, Mary S, Brazo P, Dollfus S. Psychiatric manifestations of vitamin B12 deficiency: a case report. *L'Encephale* 2003; 29(6):560–5.

18 Metzler D, Miller WH, Edwards CS . Psychiatric manifestations of vitamin B-12 deficiency: an update. http://jdc.jefferson.edu/cgi/viewcontent.cgi?article=1287&context=jeffjpsychiatry (Accessed 8 April 2015).

19 NHS Choices. Clinical depression. http://www.nhs.uk/conditions/depression/Pages/Introduction.aspx (Accessed 29 April 2015).

20 Bolander-Gouaille CA. Treatment of depression: time to consider folic acid and vitamin B12. *Journal of Psychopharmacology* 2005; 19: 59–6.

21 Ramsey D, Muskin P. Vitamin deficiencies and mental health: How are they linked? *Current Psychiatry* 2013; 12(01): 37-44.

22 Ibid.

23 Roberts SH, Bedson E, Tranter R. Half-baked? B vitamins and depression. *American Journal of Clinical Nutrition* 2010; 92: 269–270.

Chapter 7

Living with pernicious anaemia

Potential impact on lifestyle

We have seen in previous chapters that some patients who have pernicious anaemia experience none of the symptoms associated with the disease, while some others suffer only mild symptoms that disappear once replacement therapy injections of B_{12} have been started. (Whilst these patients will require treatment for the rest of their lives, the disease will have little or no impact on their everyday lives.) Others find that they have to make slight adjustments to their lifestyle in order to cope with their condition; many, however, find that their symptoms do not get much better and the impact of these can result in marital strife, the ending of relationships, termination of careers and even children being taken into care; I know this because I deal with these occurrences on a daily basis.

Certainly there are some members of the Pernicious Anaemia Society who are free of symptoms, but these are in the minority, as might be expected; those who are symptom-free do not have much motivation to join the Society, until perhaps their supplement therapy is scaled down or even stopped (see page 130). Most of the (at the time of writing) 7,000+ members of the Society have had to make adjustments to their lives in order to better manage their condition.

In this respect patients joining the Pernicious Anaemia Society tend to do so as a 'distress purchase' – they are desperate to find advice on how to manage their condition and turn to the Society for help.

My lack of a scientific background means that I often struggle to answer questions on the complex biochemistry that is involved in understanding pernicious anaemia, but when it comes to how the disease affects the everyday lives of patients I'm on much firmer ground. Every day an average of 10 telephone enquiries are made to the offices of the Pernicious Anaemia Society, and the vast majority of them are routed through to me. Every day I deal with often traumatised patients who are having problems dealing with the illness, even though they have received a firm diagnosis and are having their B$_{12}$ deficiency addressed. As we have seen from the case studies in the chapters so far, these problems can even include people being 'sectioned' as mentally unfit just because they are not receiving the correct treatment, with all the attendant distress that brings for them, their friends and family.

From all these calls, I know how the disease affects patients' well-being, their career and work, their family and friends and a host of other issues. I also know from personal experience how difficult this can be, so in this chapter I will try and summarise the advice that the Pernicious Anaemia Society tries to provide to callers and members on these real-life issues. (There is more detail on this in my earlier book, *Living with Pernicious Anaemia and Vitamin B$_{12}$ Deficiency*.)

Developing a coping strategy

A common enquiry to the offices of the Pernicious Anaemia Society is from patients still experiencing the symptoms of pernicious anaemia after treatment has commenced – they want to know 'when will I feel better?' I have to respond by stating that unfortunately some patients will remain symptomatic after treatment has begun, regardless of how often they are treated. Often the caller will not be the patient but a family member or friend who will have noticed the patient struggling to keep up with domestic tasks, work commitments or both.

I sometimes advise that perhaps he or she needs more frequent treatment, mention the sub-lingual spray and other alternative delivery methods and suggest that the patient discusses additional supplementation with his or her doctor and when this avenue has been explored to call again. Sometimes, though this is very rare, the caller will telephone again and report that the additional supplementation has made a tremendous difference and that he or she has been able to live their lives as they did before they developed the disease, but more likely that patient will report that he or she still feels dreadful and is struggling to live a normal life.

There's little more I can do than to offer sympathy and suggest that the patient needs to develop a coping strategy to best manage his or her condition. A coping strategy can mean making small, hardly noticeable changes to everyday life, such as going to bed earlier to ensure adequate sleep, or it might mean making life-changing decisions that can involve a change of job or a new career. These changes are likely to affect family and social life, careers and education.

Family and social life

Patients who are still symptomatic after treatment has begun will notice that their family and social life will be affected to some degree. This can range from the family joking about the patient's memory problems, to the termination of long-term relationships or marriages and everything in between. The worst cases involve children. Where the family and partners are able to make allowances for the patient's needs, the family unit can simply make slight adjustments to their routine and carry on with their lives. Unfortunately, I am aware of numerous cases where the patient's coping strategy has left the partner unable to make a commitment to the relationship and the patient is not able to count on any close support to help him or her manage the condition. One of the issues involved here is one not often talked about – loss of libido. When a patient is struggling with incessant fatigue and straining to cope with everyday tasks it shouldn't come as a surprise that the relationship founders when it comes to sex.

However, it is the patient's social life that causes the greatest strain in many cases. The need for long periods of sleep may mean that the patient needs to retire to bed in the early evening, or even very early evening, which means that social activities that are usually enjoyed during the latter part of the day become non-existent. This leads the patient's partner to attend any social gatherings, family occasions and other activities alone which, in many cases is not a problem. However, it can cause resentment, especially when other sufferers, who might be family members, experience none of the ongoing symptoms and do not have to make any adjustments to their life.

It is often difficult for the patient's partner to understand just how profoundly pernicious anaemia can affect sufferers' lives and I have been asked by patients on numerous occastions to speak with their partner to explain what is going on. Strangely enough, when members of the Pernicious Anaemia Society hold social events (always, by the way, during the morning), it is not only members of the Society who swap stories, experiences and advice, but also the partners of those patients and, just as the patients feel a sense of relief that their experiences are shared by others, so too do their partners who receive and offer sympathy to others in a similar position to themselves.

Careers

It isn't often that a day passes without someone telephoning the offices of the Pernicious Anaemia Society seeking advice about work-related issues. These calls always involve patients who have been diagnosed and are being treated but who are still symptomatic to some degree or other. Sometimes the patient is just seeking reassurance that he or she is not imagining that they are still experiencing the symptoms, while others are in a desperate fight to carry on with their work and want advice relating to their legal position. In the worst cases, careers are brought to an untimely end and years of hard work and dedication will have been for nothing. These problems centre on the fact that people with pernicious anaemia can still experience the worst symptoms of the condition even after treatment has begun, though just how severe the symptoms are and how they affect the individual's ability to carry out his or her workplace activities will vary from patient to patient. Bosses and colleagues generally do not understand this and assume that with diagnosis and treatment everything should be back to normal.

One week in late 2014 I found myself offering advice and support to five members of the Pernicious Anaemia Society who were having problems with their careers and having to negotiate with their employer to make allowances for their still ongoing symptoms; the five involved were a long-haul airline pilot, two firearms officers in the same police force (they were husband and wife actually), an architect and a primary school teacher. All five, unfortunately, were forced to abandon their careers because their employers couldn't make the necessary adjustments to allow them to continue with their careers.

Many of the callers ask whether pernicious anaemia is classed as a disability. It isn't unless the patient has been diagnosed as having 'sub-acute combined degeneration of the cord secondary to pernicious anaemia' (see Chapter 6). It used to be the case that in the UK local authorities kept a register of disabled people in their respective areas; however, this no longer always happens though some authorities continue to operate this scheme – Hampshire does, for example. Individuals applying for a 'blue badge' for parking are individually assessed, with the main qualification being that the applicant is receiving the higher mobility rate of the disability living allowance (DLA) or meets the 'moving around' or 'planning and following journeys' descriptors of the newly introduced 'personal independence payment' (PIP).

In the UK the rights of disabled people are now set out in the Equality Act of 2010 which replaced the older Disability Discrimination Act of 1995. This newer act, like its predecessor states quite clearly (just like the United Nations Convention on Disability) that, should any employee see their health deteriorate to the extent that he or she is disabled, then the employer has the duty to make 'reasonable adjustments' so the employee is not disadvantaged compared with non-disabled employees. The UK's Gov.uk website provides a definition of what constitutes a disability:

> You're disabled under the Equality Act 2010 if you have a
> physical or mental impairment that has a 'substantial' and
> 'long-term' negative effect on your ability to do normal daily
> activities.[1]

If an individual has been diagnosed as having sub-acute combined degeneration of the cord secondary to pernicious anaemia that can mean that he or she can be said to be disabled – I am, for example. However, patients with pernicious anaemia who are still symptomatic after treatment has begun will *not* be considered to be disabled. And this means that, just like those five unlucky members of the Pernicious Anaemia Society that I mentioned above, their employers are not obliged to make 'reasonable adjustments' and their careers may have to end.

There are three things to note here. Firstly, until the Pernicious Anaemia Society was formed there was no vehicle by which the experiences of patients could be aired to health professionals and others. For decades it had been assumed that once treatment had commenced, patients' symptoms would disappear (and, of course, in some cases that is exactly what does happen). The Society, however, is aware that a total or partial alleviation of symptoms does not occur in all cases, and this means that the Society is in a unique position to give evidence on this matter at any future test case. Such a test case, if found in favour of a symptomatic individual with pernicious anaemia, could mean that such patients might, in the future, be regarded as having a disability – after all the definition refers to 'mental impairment' as well as physical.

Secondly, as we saw earlier in the book, it is often a long journey to a definitive diagnosis of pernicious anaemia, because the patient will often ignore or fight the symptoms for many years before they become so bad that a doctor is eventually told about them. Now, how many as yet undiagnosed sufferers of pernicious anaemia are trying to cope with the extreme tiredness, constant weariness, lack of concentration, irritability etc. *and* flying loaded aircraft around the world, pointing high-powered rifles at suspects, designing buildings and trying to teach children? And how many diagnosed patients are continuing to carry out potentially dangerous jobs less than perfectly because they know that their employer will not have to make any reasonable adjustments to their workload? Think about that when you are next on final approach to Heathrow.

Thirdly, when it comes to employment law it is important that the legal profession are aware that some patients will still experience the symptoms of pernicious anaemia after treatment has commenced in order that any employment tribunal can in turn be made aware of this issue before reaching any conclusion. That is why in 2014 I briefed four different solicitors about the ongoing symptoms and the implications for employment. Those solicitors' details can be found in Appendix 5 (page 262): all are aware of the implications of pernicious anaemia and workplace issues. Patients who have pernicious anaemia and are still symptomatic are not, at the time of writing, considered to have a disability of any kind, but that doesn't mean that they will never be considered so.

Education

Just as patients who are still symptomatic often struggle to cope with the demands of their job, so too will still-symptomatic students find that their education becomes increasingly difficult to manage. Contrary to what is popularly believed, pernicious anaemia does not only affect elderly people – four individuals who were under the age of 10 at the time of diagnosis responded to our survey.[i] Infantile pernicious anaemia and juvenile pernicious anaemia affect not only the social lives of young people (some very young – we have had members of the Pernicious Anaemia Society as young as 12 months), but also mean that further challenges are encountered in education. Just as employers are unaware that pernicious anaemia can and does affect how employees carry out their work, so too are teachers unaware how pernicious anaemia can affect children, and that children and juveniles can remain symptomatic after treatment has begun.

Again, the treatment usually prescribed in the UK of a 1 mg injection of hydroxocobalamin every three months means that sometimes the young person will start to experience the symptoms of pernicious anaemia long before his or her next injection is due. Also, some young people won't be aware that perhaps they need more frequent injections and will suffer in silence while struggling to keep up with classmates.

---

[i] The survey found that 'The ages of respondents at the time of diagnosis of pernicious anaemia varied from less than 10 years (four individuals) to greater than 80 years (12 individuals). The most frequent age at diagnosis was 41–50 years (228 individuals).'

Every telephone enquiry concerning young people under the age of 16 that has been made to the offices of the Pernicious Anaemia Society has been made by grandmothers who notice a deterioration in their grandchild in the run-up to the next injection – sometimes that deterioration can be many weeks before the next injection is due and will involve mood changes that lead to non-cooperation in class work, sullen demeanour and irritability. The family's doctor will not prescribe more frequent injections believing, as most doctors do, that the child's treatment is perfectly adequate. The family and teachers trust the doctor's opinion and, unfortunately, that's when educational psychologists often get involved, and the child is labelled as having 'behavioural problems'. And whilst adults are able to find a doctor who will treat them according to their need, or can purchase more B_{12} in some form or other in order to feel better, these options are not available to children unless their parents understand the issues.

Juvenile pernicious anaemia can mean that the sufferer forgoes the joys and pleasures of growing up and is left feeling bewildered, confused and resentful. Thankfully I have only had to deal with cases of infantile and juvenile pernicious anaemia very rarely – perhaps three times a year. All that I can do is provide teachers and parents with a statement that says that, unfortunately, and for reasons that remain unknown, some patients with pernicious anaemia remain symptomatic once their B_{12} deficiency has been corrected. This can lead to schools and colleges making some allowances for the patient in exams etc, but there's not a lot more that can be done and I know of several instances where students in further and higher education have left their course because of their condition. When I encounter these situations, at the back of my mind is the niggling question of whether these issues could be addressed by simply increasing the frequency of the patient's replacement therapy injections of B_{12}.

Insurance

Some insurance companies charge patients with pernicious anaemia extra for travel insurance whilst others don't, so it's worth shopping around and comparing companies. Critical illness cover can be refused (which happened to me), especially if the diagnosis is subacute combined degeneration of the cord secondary to pernicious anaemia, as can life insurance – though some insurance companies do not recognise straightforward pernicious anaemia as being a higher risk factor.

Summary

As the Chairman of a patient support group for people with pernicious anaemia and their families and friends I am in a unique position to evaluate how the disease affects the everyday lives of sufferers and those close to them. It causes distress in the workplace and family strife. It can remain a debilitating disease even after treatment to rectify the B$_{12}$ deficiency has commenced, whilst on the other hand it may have no effect or consequences for patients who were non-symptomatic even before they were diagnosed, or who responded to their treatment by seeing their symptoms almost miraculously disappear. I offer no explanation for these differing responses to replacement therapy injections; rather, the purpose of this chapter, just like the work of the Pernicious Anaemia Society, is to raise awareness that pernicious anaemia affects the lives of different patients in many different ways.

Reference

1 GOV.UK. Definition of disability under the Equality Act 2010. https://www.gov.uk/definition-of-disability-under-equality-act-2010 (Accessed 14 April 2015).

Chapter 8

Current trends and future developments

This book has outlined the failings in diagnosing vitamin B_{12} deficiency and pernicious anaemia. As we have seen, there are issues surrounding what constitutes a deficiency, how B_{12} is measured and what form of of the vitamin should be measured. In addition, there are then problems with identifying whether any deficit in the vitamin is due to lack of intrinsic factor, which would lead to a diagnosis of pernicious anaemia. Similarly, there are problems with some, though not all, patients getting treated according to their individual need. Whilst these issues are now being acknowledged by a growing number of medical professionals, it is widely thought that nothing is being done to address these problems. Social media in particular is awash with negative views and comments on individual doctors and the medical profession in general. Contrary to these negative views, a great deal of investigation is taking place into these issue; it's just that these studies are not in the public eye, not least because the investigators are, quite rightly, jealously guarding their work until the results of their experiments are ready to be published, and then reviewed and analysed by other professionals.

These problems with the diagnosis and treatment of pernicious anaemia (and let's remember that the biggest cause of vitamin B_{12}

deficiency is pernicious anaemia) have probably existed for decades, but until the Pernicious Anaemia Society came into being there was no single channel whereby any discontent could be brought to the attention of medical professionals and decision-makers. Remember that when I set up the Pernicious Anaemia Society my sole intention was to provide newly diagnosed patients, along with their families and friends, with a plain-English explanation of their medical condition because such information was not available when I was diagnosed. The original online forum soon became a repository for hundreds of stories of misdiagnosis and under-treatment, which is why the Society became a registered charity with specific aims and objectives, the main one being to raise awareness of the problems with diagnosis and treatment amongst the medical profession. And that is what we, as a Society, have been doing for the past eight years, with, I like to think, some success. We have been successful in pushing the issues that we have identified on to the political and, more importantly, health agendas; that has taken tact, diplomacy and buckets full of patience – as a representative of a patient group I am an outsider as far as the medical profession is concerned.

Ideas are seldom just one single entity but a combination of different concepts that come together to form something new. Medicinal knowledge is based on ideas from chemistry, biochemistry, mathematics, physics, psychology and a whole host of other sources, but sometimes not all the ingredients are present or available. The medical ideas about pernicious anaemia for decades missed one important input – that of patients. It is the Pernicious Anaemia Society that has articulated the experiences of patients and corrected this imbalance. However, that doesn't mean that everything is now as it should be. The issues that we have raised have challenged long-established protocols and beliefs and our experiences and findings will have to be investigated fully before any changes are made. Medicine is based on scientific explanations of different phenomena and those explanations have to be subject to 'peer review' – criticism and analysis from fellow professionals – before finally being accepted. That said, there have been some promising developments in the past year and it is to these developments that we now turn.

Developments in diagnosing B$_{12}$ deficiency

Back in Chapter 3 we looked at the problems with assessing B$_{12}$ status owing to the shortcomings of the currently used serum B$_{12}$ test. We also reviewed some seemingly better tests that might give a more accurate picture of the B$_{12}$ status of patients. When a patient has low B$_{12}$ his or her total homocysteine (tHcy) level is raised, along with his/her level of methylmalonic acid (MMA), and while tests for both these substances are acknowledged to be better than the current B$_{12}$ test, they are not widely available and they are expensive. Here's what the new BCSH guidelines (see page xvi) say:

> Plasma tHcy and/or plasma MMA, depending on availability, may be considered as supplementary tests to determine biochemical cobalamin deficiency in the presence of clinical suspicion of deficiency but an indeterminate serum cobalamin level.

There is also the 'active B$_{12}$' issue where instead of measuring the total amount of B$_{12}$ in the patient's blood only the active B$_{12}$ is measured – holotranscobalamin (HoloTC). Remember that up to 90% of a patient's B$_{12}$ could be the inactive type (holohaptocorrin) which doesn't play any part in the biological process. Well, a group of scientists, all with a deep interest in all things to do with B$_{12}$, have come up with a model that is based on some very complex and clever mathematics, which means that if they know the serum B$_{12}$ figure they can accurately predict the patient's MMA and tHcy, along with the patient's HoloTC.[1]

The researchers say:

> We provide equations and spreadsheets that combine two,
> three or four biomarkers into one diagnostic parameter
> called the 'combined indicator of vitamin B 12 status'.
> Adjustment of this indicator is required at serum or plasma
> folate < 10 nmol/l because of increase in tHcy.

So, through an extremely clever use of mathematical formulae, the test result of the suspect B$_{12}$ test can be 'translated' or converted into what the other three more reliable tests would have produced. And that's not all. The team also addressed another contentious issue – the cut-off figure to determine any deficiency: 'Revised cut-points and guidelines for the novel approach are suggested.' The combined indicator is also able to measure folate.

I don't know how long this multinational team[i] worked on this project but it was likely to have been many years. So what, you might be wondering, happens now? Well, the paper has been published and now it will undergo serious scrutiny by other scientists. It'll be analysed carefully, the calculations checked and double-checked and will generally be 'pulled apart' and critiqued. If the research stands up to that scrutiny, the new indicator may eventually be adopted by health services around the globe, but only if it can be proved that the current system is seriously flawed. This is where the Pernicious Anaemia Society can play a part – by raising awareness of how the current (flawed) test is affecting patients' lives. It is still early days for this new combined indicator of B$_{12}$ status, and it may or may not be adopted, but it is an important step forward on the journey to better diagnostic tests.

[i] They come from Aarhus University in Denmark, the University of Davis in California, USA, and Rutgers University in New Jersey, USA.

Hand-held B_{12} monitors

There's another test that's been developed which I attended a presentation about. Again, the mathematics are very complex but this test has already been developed and is currently being evaluated. Early results are that it is a much better indicator of the B_{12} status than the test currently being used. There are large sums of money involved here and the developers are keen to keep their work as low-key as possible and so I've been asked not to give out the exact details. What I can say, however, is that this device, whilst still the size of a table at the time of writing, is being scaled down so that it can become a hand-held device that doctors can use to instantly get a picture of the patient's B_{12} status. The developers gave me this statement: 'We are working towards tracking vitamin B_{12} and associated compounds in humans in an efficient and cost-effective system that is, ultimately, suitable for a hand-held monitoring device.' This really is an exciting development.

Active B_{12} test

Another development which the authors of the new BCSH guidelines believe offers hope for better diagnosis of low B_{12} is the 'Active-B_{12}', or holotranscobalamin (HoloTC), test. The guidelines say: 'HoloTC is suggested as a suitable assay for assessment of cobalamin status in a routine diagnostic laboratory in the future.'

As I mentioned in Chapter 3, the current test measures the total amount of B_{12} in the blood serum. The test for HoloTC measures only the 'active' B_{12} in the blood, differentiating between active and inactive forms. It is only the active form of B_{12} that plays a part in biological processes.[ii]

[ii] The 'inactive' form of B_{12} is called holohaptocorrin.

The HoloTC test is gradually being introduced in several countries. There is, however, a great deal of misunderstanding about its introduction. To be clear, there are four major manufacturers of the machines currently used to measure, or fail to measure, *total* B$_{12}$. while, as Dr Ralph Carmel has said: 'Axis-Shield Diagnostics is the only manufacturer to offer the Active-B$_{12}$ test.' Here's what Axis-Shield Diagnostics told me in a statement:

> Blood testing in hospital and private laboratories is highly automated and the market is dominated by four major medical diagnostic companies, each with their own different automated instruments. Each manufacturer has control over which tests can or cannot be performed on their respective instruments. All of the four big players have total vitamin B12 tests available on their own instruments but not all have Active-B12. At Axis-Shield, we recognised that Active-B12 offers a number of important advantages over Total B12 so we have developed, or are developing, the Active-B12 test for use on these instruments.

This indicates they don't want to be the only player to offer the active B$_{12}$ test but to see the other manufacturers modify their machines to incorporate this test also:

> A key part of our strategy to convince the manufacturers to include Active-B12 in their test portfolio is to present the benefits that Active-B12 can offer, including testimonials from laboratories that already offer the test as well as case studies from patients where the Total B12 test has failed to diagnose a vitamin B12 deficiency.

So far, so good, but I can hear you asking how long before we can expect the current total B$_{12}$ test to be replaced by the new active-B$_{12}$ one? Axis-Shield said:

Our aim is to have Active-B12 available from all four major diagnostic companies by 2018 and thus allow the majority of laboratories worldwide to offer this test on a routine basis.

So, at the time of writing, we have to wait another three years before this test is widely available – these things take time. There is, however, something else to bear in mind – the new test is not without its critics as we saw back in Chapter 3. I asked Dr Dominic Harrington (who you will remember has been working with the new test for a number of years) about any shortcomings of the new Active-B$_{12}$ test. He replied:

Studies have shown that the Axis-Shield/Abbott holotranscobalamin assay has a slightly superior Receiver Operator Characteristic curve when compared with the existing assay – that is, it demonstrated superior sensitivity and specificity. However, in common with many tests used in the diagnostic laboratory, the vitamin B12 and Active-B12 assays both generate a proportion of results which are considered to be indeterminate and there is evidence emerging that transcobalamin variants of low prevalence in some populations are not recognised by the assay.

So where does that leave us in the fight to get an accurate measure of the patient's B$_{12}$ status? Dominic suggests further tests:

This inherent limitation can be addressed through further secondary testing using a functional marker of status. A functional marker of status gives an indication of vitamin B12 utilisation at the tissue level. Suitable functional markers include circulatory concentrations of methylmalonic acid and homocysteine.

The mode of application and the assignment of cut-off values for Active-B$_{12}$ are variable, i.e. some use it as a sole status indicator; others as a first line screening test in conjunction with a functional marker to evaluate indeterminate results; others as a second line test used in tandem to support indeterminate results from serum B$_{12}$ measurement. There is still a lot to learn about the new assay.

B$_{12}$ breath test

There's one final development in evaluating the B$_{12}$ status of patients and it comes from a paper published in 2011 – the development of a simple breath test known as the B$_{12}$ breath test (BBT).[2] The test is based on the metabolism of sodium propionate to carbon dioxide which involves B$_{12}$ and has shown favourable results. Here's how the researchers summed up the study:

> In this study we have developed and refined the B12 breath test to be a simple diagnostic test for B12 deficiency. Overall, these results indicate that the vitamin B12 breath test is a non-invasive, sensitive, specific, and reproducible diagnostic test to detect vitamin B12 deficiency.

And that was it! I've been unable to find out any more about this test. I don't know if the idea has been developed or is planned to be developed or whether it has just been dropped. Given what has been said in previous chapters about screening for B$_{12}$ deficiency, this non-invasive, presumably cheap yet reliable test held the promise to be an exceedingly useful tool to detect any B$_{12}$ deficiency before patients develop any serious problems associated with low status.

Now it's time to move on to developments in treating B$_{12}$ deficiency and pernicious anaemia. I will concentrate on the treatment of pernicious anaemia, as any dietary deficiency can be easily resolved by taking an oral supplement or changing diet. To that end, I would consider patients who have had an ileostomy effectively to be patients with pernicious anaemia, even though their condition is not due to autoimmune atrophic gastritis.

Developments in treating pernicious anaemia

As we saw earlier in the book, some patients report feeling better when receiving one particular form of B_{12} rather than another, and this could be due to the fact that some people are better able to convert cyanocobalamin or hydroxocobalamin into methylcobalamin. Both methylcobalamin and adenosylcobalamin are 'active' forms of B_{12} but they are quite distinct entities and play different roles in biology. Here is one explanation of the biochemistry:

> Vitamin B12 has two active forms, methylcobalamin (MeCbl) and adenosylcobalamin (AdoCbl), formed as a result of two distinct metabolic cascades. Their metabolic fates and thereby their functions are also distinct. AdoCbl is the major form in cellular tissues stored in the mitochondria. MeCbl is found in the cytosol, and it predominates in blood and in other body fluids.[3]

Whilst methylcobalamin is readily available as an injection, adenosylcobalamin isn't, which raises the question of whether some patients might see a total alleviation of their symptoms if they received adenosylcobalamin instead of the inactive forms of the vitamin or methylcobalamin. It's time to examine this particular form of B_{12}.

Adenosylcobalamin

Adenosylcobalamin is relatively unstable, and is especially prone to degradation in bright light. It can be thought of as one of the purest forms of naturally occurring B_{12}, as this is the B_{12} compound that most bacteria make. (Remember, only bacteria have the ability to make this micronutrient.) Most commercial B$_{12}$ is extracted from bacteria after the bacteria have been treated with cyanide. This produces cyanocobalamin, which can then be purified in organic solvent and has the advantage that it is not light-sensitive. However, in recent years it has become easier to extract adenosylcobalamin, though at the time of writing it is still not available as an injection. (A quick internet search has, however, shown that it is readily available in liquid and tablet form online.) There is a great deal of interest in which forms of cobalamin are more readily absorbed and taken up by living systems.

Remember at this point that 10% of the Pernicious Anaemia Society use methylcobalamin, even though it isn't licensed in Europe or North America and, as we have seen, because of the enormous cost involved in getting it licensed, and the very limited financial returns involved, it is unlikely that it ever will become licensed.

Professor Martin Warren is Professor of Biochemistry and Head of the School of Biosciences at the University of Kent at Canterbury; he is also Professorial Fellow of the UK's Biotechnology and Biological Sciences Research Council. Martin and his colleagues made headlines in May 2014 when they published the results of their research that looked at how B$_{12}$ is made. Here's the press release:

> A scientific breakthrough, led by Professor of Biochemistry Martin Warren, has revealed how vitamin B12/anti-pernicious anaemia factor is made – a challenge often referred to as 'the Mount Everest' of biosynthetic problems.

> The research team hopes that this newly-acquired information can be used to help persuade bacteria to make the vitamin in larger quantities, contributing to its use, for example, in medication for people suffering with the blood disorder pernicious anaemia.

Now someone who has successfully climbed the Mount Everest of biosynthetic problems would be the one to ask whether patients who have pernicious anaemia could use adenosylcobalamin as replacement therapy B_{12} instead of cyanocobalamin, hydroxocobalamin or methylcobalamin. And so that is what I asked him, and his reply was surprising:

> Yes – they could, but it is not clear what the advantage
> would be. Cyanocobalamin is the most stable of these
> compounds; hydroxocobalamin has a tendency to break
> down and methylcobalamin, as with adenosylcobalamin, is
> light-sensitive (although slightly more stable than adenosyl-
> cobalamin). We require more data on the stability of these
> molecules during the uptake process and the integration
> of the molecules into cells. Only then will we be able to
> determine the best form of cobalamin for administration
> – and even then there is the possibility that there may be
> some variation with some patients having a preference for
> different forms.

Professor Warren's comments are fascinating because, as far as I'm aware, this is the first time there has been any acknowledgement that patients may respond better to one form of B_{12} than another – something that members of the Pernicious Anaemia Society have known for a long time.

I dug a little deeper and asked Martin, if adenosylcobalamin could be used as replacement therapy, what, if any, would the advantages be over the established treatments? He replied:

> This is where a bit more research would be handy to look
> at the relative uptake and stability of these versions of B_{12}.
> In reality we are not sure what really happens to adenosyl-
> cobalamin or methylcobalamin – do they lose their upper
> ligand (the adenosyl or methyl group) during the uptake

process? Certainly, when taken into the cell the upper ligand is removed by a protein called CblC, which also removes the cyano group from cyanocobalamin. So there is lot still to learn about the uptake of cobalamin and its movement into the cell.

Here we are, then, back to the problem of assessing the B$_{12}$ status in patients. Some patients have some or all of the symptoms of a deficiency yet their serum B$_{12}$ can be normal or even exceptionally high while others may have low levels but no symptoms. The reason could be, or probably is, due to what happens at cell level.

Then there's the problem with storing B$_{12}$; Martin went on:

> Also, we don't know a great deal about its storage – or in what form it is stored. This is significant given the fact that patients are only given B$_{12}$ shots every three months. If hydroxocobalamin is given – and it is known to break down – then cyanocobalamin or methylcobalamin may be better agents. However, it may be that hydroxocobalamin is stored as methyl or adenosylcobalamin once it is taken up. The research sounds simple but it is actually quite difficult to do as our cells contain so little of the vitamin.

So, not only do we know that some patients will probably respond better to one form of artificial B$_{12}$ rather than others, but also there may be a problem in some patients storing the vitamin – all pointers towards why some patients need more frequent injections than others.

I told Martin that 10% of members of the Pernicious Anaemia Society use unlicensed methylcobalamin and his response was quite surprising.

> The administration of methylcobalamin makes some sense – it is a natural form of B$_{12}$ that is required in humans for an

enzyme that makes and recycles an essential amino acid. It could be that methylcobalamin is absorbed into the cell and utilised immediately, and therefore could have greater efficacy than cyanocobalamin or hydroxycobalamin. However, it is light-sensitive and should be handled in a darkened room. More research is really required to explore the uptake and incorporation of these different forms of cobalamin.

It is so refreshing to talk to someone who doesn't automatically dismiss the notion that some patients respond better to one particular form of B_{12} rather than another, or that some patients might need more frequent treatment, or ascribe their responses to a 'placebo' effect.

A cure for pernicious anaemia?

It was my birthday on September 3rd, 2014 and in my daily newspaper, like most of the other dailies, there was a story of the results of a remarkable piece of research carried out by a team of scientists at the Department of Experimental Pathology at the University of Bristol in the UK.[4] The article stated that scientists had made an important breakthrough in the fight against debilitating autoimmune diseases, such as multiple sclerosis, by revealing how to stop cells attacking healthy body tissue. It went on to say that:

It's hoped this latest insight will lead to the widespread use of antigen-specific immunotherapy as a treatment for many autoimmune disorders, including multiple sclerosis (MS), type 1 diabetes, Graves' disease and systemic lupus erythematosus (SLE).

Note that there was no mention of pernicious anaemia. So, what do you think I did? That's right, two weeks later I was at the university to meet with Professor David Wraith, the lead researcher into this remarkable breakthrough, who had just had a paper published that could have a direct effect on patients with pernicious anaemia. I had a set of questions to ask him and his answers were refreshingly simple and easy to understand given the extremely complex nature of this scientific area. I began by asking him that, if he has been able to 'switch off' the gene that causes autoimmune diseases, would he be able to apply this to the anti-intrinsic factor antibody?

It would be better to say that we have learned how to 'switch off' the immune response that causes autoimmune diseases rather than the specific gene that causes disease. As I am sure you will appreciate, the immune system is complex and even the induction of antibodies against the proteins in a vaccine, for example, requires interaction between many different immune cells and the millions of genes that they each express.

Thankfully, he explained things a little further to clarify the issues:

Antibodies are made by cells derived from the bone marrow called B cells but their behaviour is controlled by another set of immune cells, T cells, which first appear in a part of the body called the thymus. To put it simply: without help from T cells the B cells can't make antibodies.

So it's all down to T cells helping out B cells when it comes to making antibodies. Antibodies are usually good things to have as they fight any invasive body. As we have seen previously, some people, like me, unfortunately produce antibodies that kill off good bodies – in my case my intrinsic factor. Consequently, I have intrinsic factor antibodies and, try as I might, over the years I have not been able to stop making them as it's beyond my control.

Before we go any further it's useful to note that an *allergen* is something the body thinks is attacking it though actually it is harmless. This may be something external, such as dust or pollen, or something internal, such as intrinsic factor;responding to it is a sort of 'friendly fire' incident. Professor Wraith continued:

> Allergy doctors have known for many years that it is possible to 'switch off' allergic responses by injecting ever-increasing doses of the allergen, usually a protein, that triggers the B cells causing the allergic response. If successful, this results in selective desensitisation of the immune system and this effectively prevents any further immune response to that specific protein. As a result, this procedure is known as antigen-specific immunotherapy. It is important to stress, however, that this is a risky business; by injecting the allergen you risk triggering a dangerous allergic response.
>
> We have developed an alternative strategy that is designed to avoid the potential side effects of antigen-specific immunotherapy. We have learned that the key cells to desensitise are T cells and we have also shown that these cells respond to small fragments of the protein known as peptides. Luckily B cells are unlikely to respond to these fragments. So, by injecting peptides rather than proteins, we can desensitise T cells without running the risk of activating disease-associated B cells.

So what has this to do with autoimmune diseases?

> In recent years we and others have shown that peptide immunotherapy can be used to prevent and treat a wide range of allergic and autoimmune diseases. This has proven highly successful in experimental models of autoimmune disease and has, more recently, been tested in clinical trials in patients with autoimmune diseases such as multiple sclerosis and systemic lupus erythematosus.

This is about as simple an explanation as I could get. It is an incredibly complex area and it left me wishing I had put a little more effort into my O-level chemistry and biology lessons (Grade U – 'unclassified' – in both). Now this chemistry and biochemistry is all very well, but could Professor Wraith apply this knowledge to switching off the immune response to intrinsic factor (IF)? After all that's what patients with pernicious anaemia will be concerned about:

> Well yes, this would be possible; however, the question is whether anti-IF antibodies are the key target for this disease. I would argue that we should be targeting the T cells specific for the major parietal cell antigen (PCA). It is, after all, the destruction of these cells that causes the reduction in IF and this lies at the heart of the disease.

This is getting right down to the source of the problem – the parietal cells. This was exciting stuff and so, probably like you, I wanted to know when this 'treatment' would be available. The answer was brilliantly simple:

> For us to design therapeutic peptides specific for PCA we will need to follow three steps:
>
> 1. produce enough PCA to allow us to screen patients with autoimmune gastritis;
>
> 2. screen a broad group of patients to confirm the importance of PCA-specific T cells; and
>
> 3. use cell lines developed from representative patients to identify potential therapeutic peptides.

Yes, yes! But how long will that take?

> If all goes well we could complete this work in two years and could then propose to use these peptides for early phase clinical trials.

Now let me get this right – would this mean then, that for the very first time there will be a *cure* for auto-immune pernicious anaemia?

If we can switch off the cells that cause damage to parietal cells then yes, it is possible that this would stop the disease in its tracks. The question is whether we could treat people early enough; can this be done before too much damage has been done to their parietal cells?

So now we are back to the thorny question of screening patients for B_{12} deficiency, for which a simple breath test would be extremely useful. Just before I made my way back to the car David thanked me and said, 'Do you know, until you had contacted me I hadn't even thought about pernicious anaemia – well done.'

The Pernicious Anaemia Society is now working with Professor Wraith and his team on a project to put together a research programme – it's early days yet but I'm sure we'll make good progress in this exciting area.

Finally, there is one member of the Pernicious Anaemia Society who is a senior figure in the world of biochemistry and who has come up with an amazingly simple delivery method for replacement therapy B_{12}. It will mean that patients won't even know that they are giving themselves a 'hit' of B_{12} throughout the day. This involves bypassing the stomach, with the vitamin going straight into the bloodstream. Is she going on to develop it? It couldn't be that simple – she's a scientist and is firstly going 'right back to basics' and examining what type of B_{12} is best suited for this method of delivery. It will probably take a few years before the development takes place, by which time I can only wonder what other developments will have evolved.

Summary

Medical researchers are continually expanding their knowledge of how the body works and why it sometimes doesn't. New fields of scientific knowledge are emerging and new discoveries are constantly feeding into a greater understanding of the human body. It is my job as Chairman of the Pernicious Anaemia Society to ensure that researchers, scientists and doctors are aware of the problems faced by patients with pernicious anaemia in order that these new developments can be applied to the diagnosis and treatment of the disease. That's all I can and should do – raise awareness; it is not my job to tell doctors or researchers what they should be doing; they would probably ignore me anyway. As one doctor put it recently, 'Your lack of scientific background becomes obvious,' a view with which I totally agree. However, although my lack of attention in O-level chemistry and biology might mean that I struggle to understand some of the basic scientific issues, my everyday contact with patients fighting the worst aspects of pernicious anaemia means I am ideally placed to make the scientific community aware of those problems.

References

1 Fedosov SN, Brito A, Miller JW, Green R, Allen L. Combined indicator of vitamin B 12 status: Modification for missing biomarkers and folate status and recommendations for revised cut-points. *Clinical Chemistry and Laboratory Medicine (CCLM)* 2015 (aop) doi: 10.1515/cclm-2014-0818 (Accessed January 2015).

2 Wagner D, Schatz R, Coston R, Curington C, Bolt D, Toskes PP. A new breath test to detect vitamin B-12 deficiency: a prevalent and poorly diagnosed health problem. *Journal Breath Research* 2011; 5(4): doi: 10.1088/1752-7155/5/4/046001.

3 Thakkar K, Billa G. Treatment of vitamin B12 deficiency – methylcobalamine? cyancobalamine? hydroxocobalamin? – clearing the confusion. *European Journal of Clinical Nutrition* 2015; 69(1):1–2.

4 Burton BR, Britton GJ, Fang H, Verhagen J, Smithers B, Sabatos-Peyton CA, Carney LJ, Gough J, Strobel S, Wraith DC. Sequential transcriptional changes dictate safe and effective antigen-specific immunotherapy. *Nature Communications* 2014; 4741 doi:10.1038/ncomms5741 (Accessed 15 June 2015).

Epilogue

It's been 10 years since I started the Pernicious Anaemia Society with the sole aim of providing newly diagnosed patients, and their families and friends, with a plain-English explanation of their newly acquired medical condition. I did this because, when I was eventually diagnosed, there was no Wikipedia, no Google and no support group for patients. An internet search on pernicious anaemia turned up some old research papers that were gobbledegook to me and, because I was still symptomatic even after my loading doses and had been left with a permanent disability, I was forced into early retirement after 20 years of teaching in further and higher education. Eventually, I managed to piece together the nature of my condition and, in one eureka moment, decided that I would start a small society that would provide patients with some support in the form of an easy-to-understand explanation of the disease.

As soon as the online forum went live it began to become clear that there were serious problems associated with both the diagnosis and treatment of pernicious anaemia. Many sufferers had waited years to find out what was wrong with them, often being told along the way that they had some other medical condition which meant that they were prescribed medicines that brought no relief but quite possibly had side effects. Consequently, these patients made repeated visits to their doctor, wasting enormous amounts of time and money before eventually being told why they were feeling so dreadful. But the journey didn't always end there, with a diagnosis and appropriate treatment. It soon became obvious that some patients needed much more frequent replacement B$_{12}$ than others, and, whereas doctors had in the past usually explained the patient's need for more injections as being a 'placebo' effect, this could no longer be so easily explained, simply because of the large numbers of patients unhappy with the one-size-fits-all regimen. They couldn't all be imagining a return of their symptoms before their next injection was due.

So, what began as a simple support group that would provide an easy-to-understand explanation of what pernicious anaemia was, soon became a campaigning pressure group with the sole aim of getting the way in which pernicious anaemia is diagnosed and treated thoroughly reviewed by someone who knows what he or she is doing – a doctor. Ten years on that remains the single objective of the Society; yes, we do our best to offer support and advice, but the main focus of the Pernicious Anaemia Society is to get the way in which the disease is diagnosed and treated reviewed.

Back in the early days the Society floundered. We lacked credibility and were regarded by medical professionals as being slightly cranky – after all, as far as they were concerned, the diagnosis and treatment of pernicious anaemia had been addressed in the early 1960s when artificial B$_{12}$ was used as a cheap and effective treatment once a diagnosis based on the Schilling test had been made. It became clear that in order to be listened to we had to be credible, and that meant that we must operate by observing long-established protocols and procedures. It meant that we, as a society, should not go around waving our arms in the air shouting 'unfair', because if we did, then nobody would take notice of us. This is something that a senior figure in the National Institute for Health and Care Excellence

(NICE) repeated to me a year or so ago. Instead, what we needed to do was provide doctors and other health professionals with the building blocks of their profession – scientific evidence. Just as a court of law doesn't accept anecdotal evidence, neither does the medical profession. Judgements and decisions are based on careful consideration of evidence presented before them, whether by other medical professionals or not.

And so we started to gather evidence in the form of the survey of members. However, the results of the survey would not be regarded as evidence unless they were published in a reputable journal and in a format that is recognised by scientists. After a number of rejections the results were published in April 2014 and, for the first time, there was a serious piece of published research that reflected on the problems faced by patients in getting a timely and accurate diagnosis and effective treatment for their condition.

Our approach is working. Last week alone eight researchers had downloaded the paper, which means that it is being read and examined; in other words it, and we as a society, are being taken notice of. And that, from humble beginnings, is the most remarkable part of the Society's history.

We've still got a long way to go and we are competing with lots of other patient groups that are vying with each other to get the attention of the medical profession, but we have crossed a Rubicon in terms of being listened to. We 'played the game' according to the rules, which is the only way to participate in the healthcare system, in order to represent our members.

As for the issues surrounding the way in which patients are treated, we are also actively pursuing various avenues to gather admissible evidence and that involves forming relationships with researchers and building a network of contacts. We now have a 'round table' of doctors and other medical professionals who we bring together once or twice a year where we, as officers of the Pernicious Anaemia Society, simply provide the gathering with a few questions and sit back while the discussions take place. The interaction between these professionals is quite remarkable and means that we are now involved with three research projects all concentrating on the way in which we, as patients, are treated. Again, there's a long way to go, but we are on the right path. This has only happened because we have acted in a rational and diplomatic manner, observing established protocols. It means that our work is not conspicuously obvious but that doesn't mean it isn't happening.

I don't know if there is another 10 years of fight left in me. This has been a hard journey and it has also been 10 years of learning and discovering. We still face challenges, including the ever-present problem of relying on a handful of volunteers to meet the ever-increasing demands on our services. We need to employ professionals who will be able to drive the Society forward but, unfortunately, that requires writing grant applications that will compete with other charities to a limited number of grant-making bodies. And that is itself a highly skilled job which requires money; it's a vicious circle but one that hopefully we will be able to break out of in order to achieve the vision of the Society:

A world that understands the nature and consequences of pernicious anaemia.

Onwards and upwards, as they say.

Appendix 1

Martyn's story

My story starts in September 2001. The previous year I had turned 40 and I was in my 18th year of lecturing in further education. I had a very active lifestyle, running a popular National Diploma course for full-time students, and in my spare time hill walking and leading walking expeditions, playing drums in a rock band, teaching drum-kit to exam standard, and playing tennis. I was a senior examiner for A-level politics and an examiner for the Chartered Institute of Marketing's professional qualifications. I was always 'on the go'. Then around September 2001 I started to feel really tired for the first time in my life. I knew what it was like to be tired after three days of hill walking – and that was a nice tired. But this tiredness was more than physical and mental exhaustion. It was a ubiquitous and insidious tiredness that never really went away. I was even tired after a good night's sleep. Like many other people of my age, I put this strange feeling down to my reaching middle age. There were other little indicators that middle age had arrived. I started to forget things, even found concentrating to be more and more difficult, and began to experience breathlessness more and more. 'This is it,' I thought. 'It's all downhill from here.'

I still kept up my hectic lifestyle and one evening I was playing in a band at a local gig. At the end of the set, and in true rock-star fashion, I jumped off the stage onto the dance-floor below. I landed in a pool of what was probably beer and found myself suddenly horizontal about five feet above the floor before suddenly falling hard on my back. It was quite a spectacular piece of cabaret for a finale and the crowd were genuinely pleased to see me get up and laugh off the whole event. There was apparently no damage done. A few days later my legs went numb overnight. I awoke in the morning and realised that I had no feeling from my toes up to the middle of my thighs. And my feet and knees seemed to be bloated. 'Probably due to the fall,' I thought. 'They'll return to normal soon.'

They didn't. After a month or six weeks of having no feeling in my legs and feet I booked an appointment with a doctor. It was to be the first of a great many. He didn't seem particularly concerned, explaining that it was probably due to the fall but that it was best to let nature do the healing. I agreed and, reassured that everything would soon be back to normal, resumed my busy life.

The tiredness became increasingly difficult to deal with. Even as a child I had managed on the minimum amount of sleep. I remember being told by my friends' mothers not to knock on their doors before nine o'clock, which meant that for three hours in the mornings I had to occupy myself alone. I can remember thinking it quite unremarkable that Mrs Thatcher needed just four hours' sleep per night. And here I was, having to force myself awake every morning. The breathlessness was bizarre as it seemed to require me to yawn and yawn and yawn as well as take deep breaths one after another. Then my concentration took a dive and I started to have 'fogs'. These are quite difficult to explain to somebody who hasn't experienced them, but it is as if there is a 'fog' that prevents you from understanding things clearly; it's as if something is between you and what you are looking at or hearing or saying. These 'fogs' would last a day, or two, or three. Then I would awake one morning and suddenly everything would be clear again.

By January 2002 my legs had not repaired and I was now starting to stumble and had developed an ungainly gait – I was walking like Herman Munster. This was around the time that I suddenly became aware that I could not tolerate heights and would become very unsteady on my feet when looking up. There was obviously something wrong and one of the doctors at my local surgery sent me to a neurosurgeon for a consultation. 'Well, you had a fall; you got back up – I don't think this is related to the fall,' he said. 'I want you to have an MRI scan to rule out a number of things.' 'What's an MRI scan?' I asked blankly. He explained that MRI stood for 'magnetic resonance imaging', and that it might be able to explain the numbness and unusual gait that I had developed. I went ahead with the scan, which proved that there was 'nothing sinister there'. (I later discovered that he thought I might have cancer of the spinal cord.)

Whilst all of this was going on I was still carrying out my normal hectic schedule and discovering new things wrong with me. In Dublin, with a mini-bus full of students, I stopped to ask the way of two Gardai who were walking away from me. I went to run after them, but discovered it was impossible. My legs just wouldn't go fast enough and I made quite a spectacle for the unsympathetic students, who genuinely couldn't see the serious side of what might be going on. I laughed off the incident along with them, but inside I knew that my condition was deteriorating.

In the spring of 2002 I started to have personality changes. I became very irritable with students who sought help or clarification about something. And this was the part of my job that I loved the most – helping people. Now I would treat students as an irritant, and my mood swings were being noticed at home, where I was increasingly short with my wife. It was around this time that I would completely forget a conversation I had had the day before, forget where I had parked my car, get confused trying to write sentences and really just wanted to crawl into a dark hole and sleep. One day, as I left a lecture room I couldn't remember what I had talked about for the past hour before going into another lecture to talk about something for another hour – I didn't know what was happening to me. I started to experience the need to cry for no apparent reason. And I began to realise that I must be depressed. Something would have to be done, but time and time again people would listen to my symptoms and laugh it off as being middle-age related. I tried to laugh with them but was starting to get seriously worried. I didn't mention the severity of my difficulty trying to cope with everyday life to anyone, not even to any doctor. I thought that the depression was of my own making, and that the physical symptoms were all related to the fall. The tiredness, or rather the chronic fatigue, was all due to middle age – a fact confirmed by others that I talked to.

By mid-May I was close to collapse and, when walking to my local surgery for yet another doctor's appointment, I stumbled, fell in the middle of the road and couldn't get up. I know how it feels to be ridiculed and scorned for being drunk in the middle of the day because as I tried to get up onlookers thought that I was completely inebriated. A police officer eventually helped me to my feet and I convinced him that I was not drunk. 'What's wrong with you?' he asked sympathetically. 'I don't know,' I replied. The police officer and his colleague kindly took me home in their car – the first and last time I have ever been in a police car. I was confused, frustrated, angry and very, very, very tired. After an hour or so I telephoned my sister. She is additionally a sister in that she is a nursing sister in the community – what used to be called a district nurse. She immediately drove to my house where I was stumbling around holding onto anything that was solid to help me walk. She could see that I was in some distress. My main concern was that I had not attended the appointment with the doctor. 'This is ridiculous,' she commented. 'I'm taking blood so that we can get to the bottom of this.' At least that's what I seem to remember. This was not a normal fog that I was in – this was a real 'pea-souper', with no sign of it lifting. I was the most needle-phobic man on the planet. I would wince at even the thought of a needle, but now I didn't care what she did and where she stuck the needle – I was just not interested. I wanted to sleep.

I can't remember much after she took the blood samples. I can't remember what conversation I had with my wife that evening, and I can't remember how I got to work the next day. But I do know that I was in a lecture room the next day because someone from personnel popped her head around the door and asked me if she could have a word with me. I stepped out of the classroom and she told me that my doctor had been on the 'phone and that I was to telephone him immediately. They had tried to call me at home, but they had my old number. I went to go back into the class, fully intending to talk what must have been drivel until the end of the lesson. She grabbed my arm. 'I think you ought to telephone him now. He seemed quite concerned.' I went into my work-room. There was nobody else in there as the other staff were all teaching. I telephoned the surgery and asked to be put through to this particular doctor.

'Are you okay?' asked the doctor, who was Irish.

'Yeah,' I lied.

'You need to come to the surgery right now. We have a diagnosis,' he said.

'What is it?'

'I'll explain when you get here. Come straight to my room.'

'I'll come now. How long will I be? I have a class at 12.'

'You'll not be doing any teaching for a while,' he replied. 'At least a week, maybe longer.'

I put the telephone down and went to see my Head of School to explain, or rather not explain, what had happened. She reassured me that there was no problem, but I could already see that I was causing headaches and difficulties. I stumbled to the doctor's surgery and went straight to his room as instructed. I can't remember how I felt. I must have been relieved that at last I had a diagnosis. And I must have been worried as to what that diagnosis would be. But everything was just too much to think about, and I was desperate for any help that I could receive. At the back of my mind must have been the knowledge that this was the only doctor in the practice that I hadn't seen before.

'We think it's sub-acute combined degeneration of the spinal cord secondary to pernicious anaemia,' he said.

I was stunned.

'Can you cure it?'

I remember this bit. I was looking straight into the doctor's face. He looked away. He looked down and to his right.

'We can sort you out. We will sort you out. It'll all be sorted.'

'What will happen?'

'You'll have to go into hospital. You'll have to have blood transfusions. We'll get you in today.'

'How long will I be in hospital?'

'We don't know.'

'A day? Two days? Three?'

'We don't know – maybe a lot longer than that.'

'A week?'

'We don't know.'

'But you can cure me?'

'We'll sort you out.'

'How long will it take to cure?'

'Well, you'll be on injections for life.'

'What kind of injections?'

'Vitamin B_{12} injections. You'll need lots in the next month and then every three months for life.'

'What do I do now?'

'You go home and wait for me to telephone you. Make sure that you give your correct number to reception and let me have it right now.'

'Can you write down what my diagnosis is?'

'Sure.' He wrote down the diagnosis on a slither of paper that advertised some medicine and I stumbled out of the room. I returned home and waited. My sister was on her way to France and I phoned her mobile. I told her the diagnosis. 'Oh, my God,' was the unhelpful response.

'I have to go into hospital for transfusions,' I told her. 'What am I going to do?'

'Well, you just have to be brave,' she replied in her best 'pull yourself together' tone of voice. I am not a hospital brave; I am a hospital wimp.

I was now very, very confused, tired, exhausted, overwhelmed and unsure what I should do. I didn't know how to react. My emotions were completely out of control and I struggled to be logical. The doctor phoned. There was no need after all to go into hospital.

'Just report to the nurse in the morning for the first of your injections,' he said.

I went to bed at three o'clock and slept solidly until eight the next day. I tried to explain things to my wife, but this was difficult. Surely my condition couldn't be due to a vitamin – you could buy vitamins on the high street. This had to be more serious than the lack of a vitamin. I had stuck the piece of paper on which the doctor had written the diagnosis to the fridge using a magnet. 'Why don't you look it up?' my wife said the next morning. I reached for a dictionary. The root cause was pernicious anaemia – the sub-acute thing was secondary to that and so I looked up 'pernicious' in the dictionary. I knew it didn't mean anything nice, but when I saw that the dictionary stated it meant not only 'ruinous' and 'destructive' but, more worryingly, 'fatal', I closed the book.

I reported to the nurse an hour later in an even more confused state than before.

'Do many people have pernicious anaemia?' I asked.

'Not many young people like you, and not many males. It's usually elderly ladies that have it.'

'Do they live long?'

'Oh yes – people used to die of it, but now we've got this.' She held up a small bottle with some reassuring red liquid in it.

'Is that the B$_{12}$?'

'Yup.'

I looked at the floor when she reached for the syringe and needle.

'Now, the secret is to relax.'

I couldn't relax. I felt a dull ache as the liquid entered my right arm muscle.

'Well done,' she said.

I now know that this isn't the easiest of injections to carry out painlessly. I have heard stories of some patients who have not driven for three months because of the pain of the injection. My first injection was pretty straightforward.

'There – see you tomorrow,' said the nurse.

'How many do I need?'

'Ummmmm,' she consulted some form. 'Doc says every day for a week, then weekly for four weeks, and then monthly for three months, then once every three months for life.'

After three days of injections the pins and needles that I had been experiencing for a year in the tips of my fingers disappeared. After a week, the fog started to clear. After a month I felt that I could cope with life for the first time in two years. I felt confident that improvements would continue.

After the last of my monthly injections I was looking forward to three months of not having one. My physical problems had not improved. My legs were still totally numb from my thighs down to my toes. I still couldn't run, my balance was awful and I found it difficult walking down stairs, but mentally I had become more focused and the fog had lifted. I could handle the physical problems and believed the mental issues would eventually fade away.

I believed that the B_{12} injections had cured me. I was wrong. I now know that there is no cure for pernicious anaemia and that the injections are just a way of keeping me alive. They contain B$_{12}$ that replaces the B$_{12}$ that I should be absorbing from my food. They keep me alive, but they don't cure me.

Six weeks after my last monthly injection I started to feel foggy again. The old symptoms returned with a vengeance. I would talk mumbo-jumbo, state facts that were obvious ('The Queen Mother has died,' I told my wife one day. 'I hope she is dead,' she replied, 'they buried her nine months ago.'); the forgetfulness returned. I became irritable and angry. I suffered severe mood swings. I couldn't cope with work. I panicked. It was all going horribly wrong again. I went back to the doctor's and found the GP who had first made the diagnosis had left the practice.

'I need another injection,' I told the senior partner in the surgery. He sat looking at me – looking at me with intensity; looking at me as if he was examining me; looking at me as if he was searching for signs of any unusual mannerisms. After a few seconds considering my request he said in a quiet voice, 'But you don't need one – every three months is the norm.'

'Perhaps for some people, but not for me,' I argued.

He gently shook his head and I thought he started to smile.

'It's all in your head,' he said. 'Would you like some antidepressants?'

'It's not in my head. I'm going back to how I was.'

'But you have more B$_{12}$ in your blood than I do,' he said.

'Doc, I know I am going back to how I was, and I don't want to go there. I'm sure another injection would stop it,' I pleaded.

'If I do a blood test it will show that you are practically swimming in B$_{12}$,' he said. 'I am only allowed to give you an injection every three months. Lots of patients believe they need more frequent injections, but we know that they don't and that they are imagining it all.'

I remember just staring at him with a completely blank expression. He stared back. After a few seconds he spoke.

'What if we send you to a haematologist – a blood specialist?'

'No problem,' I said.

A few days later I was in the consulting room of a haematologist who took blood and carried out a full physical examination.

'I need more regular injections,' I pleaded, 'and the doctors won't give me more frequent jabs, but I know, I really know, that I need them.'

'Okay,' he said.

I was speechless. Here was a consultant haematologist who knew far more about blood than the average GP and he was listening to me. I breathed a sigh of relief. It was as if a huge weight had been lifted from my shoulders.

'But why won't they prescribe more frequent jabs?' I asked this angel of a man.

'Because for most people an injection every three months is fine, and the guidelines they follow state three-monthly injections are the norm. But we haematologists know that some people need them more often. Maybe about 18% of people with pernicious anaemia need more regular injections even though the amount of B_{12} in their blood is very high. We simply do not know what goes on at cell level and so, because there is no possibility of overdosing on B_{12}, I'll sanction an injection every month.'

I now know that I was lucky in getting monthly injections. I also know that the 18% figure that the haematologist quoted is completely wrong. The true figure is more like 80%. In addition, I now know that the injections of B$_{12}$ used to be given every month in the 1960s and that was changed to every two months in the 1970s and then to every three months in the 1980s. I also now know that some GPs refuse to sanction more frequent injections even when told to do so by hospital consultants, whether haematologists or not.

The frequency of injections remains the single most common cause of concern and complaint by members of the Pernicious Anaemia Society that I later went on to form.

Back in the GP's surgery I was in front of yet another GP who was reading the consultant's letter.

'I don't want you to see other doctors. Let me monitor this,' he said. 'This is very interesting.' He smiled at me. 'How often do you want them?'

'I don't know – but I know I can't last three months.' I said. 'My sister will give them to me,' I added.

'Well, what if I write you out a prescription and you keep the ampoules in the fridge – then your sister can give them to you whenever you want?'

'Joy,' I thought.

'That sounds a good idea,' I said.

'This is most unusual,' he said in a friendly manner. 'There is a lot of stuff that we don't know about B$_{12}$,' he admitted before adding, 'Be sure to make any future appointments with me.'

At work it was the end of term and end of year. I looked forward to the coming summer months when I would get better and, hopefully, eventually return to normal. I had been on a roller-coaster for the past two years, but now that I had a diagnosis I was hopeful that after a few months all would be well again.

The college that I worked for was sympathetic and after informal negotiations it was agreed that for the coming academic year my timetable would be adjusted so that my lectures would all take place in the mornings. I was still getting tired in the afternoons and so, with my new timetable, I would be able to finish my teaching duties at 1.30 pm. My marking and lesson preparations would be completed in the mornings or the weekends. I had no evening classes timetabled. I coped for a year.

During the summer recess of 2003 I went into the college nearly every day of the six-week holiday. I had four days when I didn't go in. I used to be at my desk at around 8.30 and would leave at around 1.00 pm. I wrote out lesson plans, updated my notes and hand-outs and completed all of my admin. I had managed one year of coping with the demands of modern teaching and I was determined that I would carry on with my career. But coping was what I was doing. I didn't realise it at the time, but I had developed a coping strategy. I was still symptomatic, even though I was up to date with my injections.

I was lucky. My employers were sympathetic and had made allowances for my condition. Towards the end of the six-week holiday I was told by a senior manager at the college that other lecturers were complaining that I was able to finish at 1.30 pm every day and that, from September, I would be expected to follow a normal timetable that would include two postgraduate evening classes. I couldn't argue, but I suspected that the complaints from other lecturers were a fabrication. I knew that going back to a full day timetable with evening classes would be difficult, but I resigned myself to it.

I was in for a nasty shock. The hectic first week of induction activities was bad enough, but when the work routine began in earnest I started to make stupid mistakes. Modern teaching in further education involves more than just lesson preparation and lectures. As a course tutor I was expected to perform a host of other duties, including helping students complete university applications, organising personal tutorials, holding team meetings, recording team meetings, preparing an on-going course report and quality control paperwork, plus a great many other associated administrative tasks that I had to do. This was all part of a further education teacher's job and it was a relentless round of administration and mentoring with some very demanding students. It was hard enough when I was well, but now I was really struggling. And along with all this I was teaching two evenings a week on a postgraduate MBA programme.

I was floundering and, after one particularly demanding day and evening, realised that I could no longer cope. I was disciplined informally for my reaction to a particularly unsavoury case of bullying (yes, it does happen at college level) and made up my mind that, because of my condition, I would no longer be able to do the job I loved and I would have to stop teaching. I resolved to leave and the feeling of relief that I would no longer have to fight to complete what once seemed mere menial tasks is still with me. Looking back I really don't know how I managed to perform my duties for the two years before diagnosis and the year that followed. It makes me shudder to think of it now. Whenever I feel sorry for myself I remind myself of the alternative lifestyle that I struggled to manage.

I have since discovered that my experience was very similar to thousands and thousands of other people's and that, even now, hundreds of other people are going through the same ordeal of trying to get diagnosed quickly and treated adequately.

Appendix 2

Symptoms of vitamin B$_{12}$ deficiency

The symptoms of B$_{12}$ deficiency, whether caused by pernicious anaemia or not, are so wide-ranging that it is tempting to list what is *not* affected by the lack of the vitamin. Below is a selection of the most common symptoms experienced by members of the Pernicious Anaemia Society. Please note that patients may have some or all of these and the symptoms will vary in the intensity they are felt from individual to individual. Medical terms are given in brackets where appropriate

Commmon/early symptoms

- Shortness of breath – 'the sighs'
- Extreme fatigue – 'waking up tired'
- Brain fogs
  - Poor concentration
  - Short-term memory loss
  - Confusion – 'handbag in the fridge syndrome'
  - Forgetting the names of everyday objects and people (nominal aphasia)
- Unaccountable and sudden diarrhoea sometimes following a bout of constipation

- Clumsiness/lack of coordination
- Cracks at the corner of the mouth (angular cheilitis)
- Swollen, cracked 'beefy' tongue (glossitis)
- Brittle, flaky nails
- Dry skin – anywhere on the body
- Mood swings
  - 'Tear jags'
  - Irritability
  - Lack of patience
  - Frustration
  - Desirability for quiet, away from bright lights, noise and crowded environments.

Neurological symptoms

- Balance problems
  - Feeling dizzy or faint
  - Bumping into things – 'the shoulder bumps'
  - General unsteadiness, especially when showering or dressing
  - Inability to stand up with eyes closed in the dark
- Numbness, especially in hands and feet (peripheral neuropathy)
- Pins and needles, especially in hands and feet (paraesthesia)
- Tinnitus – ringing or screeching in one or both ears.

Other reported symptoms

- Sleep disturbance even though exhausted/inability to sleep
- Hair loss – can range from moderate to severe
- Premature greying of hair
- Poor digestion
- Burning legs and feet (Grierson-Gopalan syndrome)
- Neuropathic pain/fibromyalgia – often only on one side of the body
- Inability to cope with heights (vertigo)

- Need to look at something as a reference to compensate for balance problems
- Hypo or hyperthyroidism
- Psoriasis/eczema/acne
- Reddening of the skin around the nose and cheeks (rosacea)
- Irregular, fast or slow heartbeat (arrhythmia)
- Rheumatoid arthritis
- Sensitivity to wheat and/or wheat products (coeliac disease)
- Weak muscles leading to problems with swallowing, chewing and opening eye(s)
- White patches that develop on the skin (vitiligo)
- Psoriatic arthritis.

Appendix 3

Tests for full blood count

The full blood count (FBC) is used as a broad screening test to check for such disorders as anaemia, infection and many other diseases. It is actually a panel of tests that examines different parts of the blood and includes the following:

- **White blood cell (WBC) count** is a count of the actual number of white blood cells per volume of blood. Both increases and decreases can be significant.
- **White blood cell differential** looks at the types of white blood cells present. There are five different types of white blood cells, each with its own function in protecting us from infection. The differential classifies a person's white blood cells into each type: neutrophils (also known as PMNs or neuts), lymphocytes, monocytes, eosinophils and basophils.
- **Red blood cell (RBC) count** is a count of the actual number of red blood cells per volume of blood. Both increases and decreases can point to abnormal conditions.
- **Haemoglobin** measures the amount of oxygen-carrying protein in the blood.
- **Haematocrit** measures the amount of space red blood cells take up in the blood. It is reported as a percentage (0 to 100) or a proportion (0 to 1).

- **Platelet count** is the number of platelets in a given volume of blood. Both increases and decreases can point to bleeding or clotting disorders.
- **Mean platelet volume (MPV)** is a machine-calculated measurement of the average size of your platelets. New platelets are larger, and an increased MPV occurs when increased numbers of platelets are being produced. MPV gives your doctor information about platelet production in your bone marrow.
- **Mean corpuscular volume (MCV)** is a measurement of the average size of your RBCs. The MCV is elevated when your RBCs are larger than normal (macrocytic), for example in anaemia caused by vitamin B$_{12}$ deficiency or folic acid deficiency. When the MCV is decreased, your RBCs are smaller than normal (microcytic), which may indicate iron-deficiency anaemia, inflammation or, occasionally, thalassaemia (inherited malformation of haemoglobin).
- **Mean corpuscular haemoglobin (MCH)** is a calculation of the amount of oxygen-carrying haemoglobin inside your RBCs. Since macrocytic RBCs are larger than either normal or microcytic RBCs, they would also tend to have higher MCH values.
- **Mean corpuscular haemoglobin concentration (MCHC)** is a calculation of the concentration of haemoglobin inside the RBCs. Decreased MCHC values (hypochromia) are seen in conditions where the haemoglobin is abnormally diluted inside the red cells, such as in iron-deficiency anaemia, long-standing inflammation or thalassaemia. Increased MCHC values (hyperchromia) are seen in conditions where the haemoglobin is abnormally concentrated inside the red cells, such as in hereditary or autoimmune spherocytosis.
- **Red cell distribution width (RDW)** is a calculation of the variation in the size of your RBCs. In some anaemias, such as iron-deficiency or pernicious anaemia, the amount of variation (anisocytosis) in RBC size (along with variation in shape – poikilocytosis) causes an increase in the RDW.

Appendix 4

Summary of new guidelines on cobalamin and folate for medical professionals

In June 2014 the British Committee for Standards in Haematology issued new, revised Guidelines on Vitamin B_{12} and Folate. The new Guidelines acknowledge the failings of the current assay used to determine B_{12} status in patients. Below are the main recommendations of the Committee:

1. The clinical picture is the most important factor in assessing the significance of test results assessing cobalamin status because there is no 'gold standard' test to define deficiency.

2. Definitive cut-off points to define clinical and subclinical deficiency states are not possible, given the variety of methodologies used and technical issues.

3. In the presence of discordance between the test result and strong clinical features of deficiency, treatment should not be delayed to avoid neurological impairment.

4. The absence of a raised MCV cannot be used to exclude the need for cobalamin testing because neurological impairment occurs with a normal MCV in 25% of cases.

5. Some assays may give false normal results in sera with high titre anti-intrinsic factor antibodies.

6. It is not entirely clear what should be regarded as a clinically normal serum cobalamin level.

7. It is even less clear what levels of serum cobalamin represent 'subclinical' deficiency.

8. Neurological symptoms due to cobalamin deficiency may occur in the presence of a normal MCV.

9. IFAB is positive in 40–60% of cases, i.e., low sensitivity, and the finding of a negative IFAB assay does not therefore rule out pernicious anaemia (hereafter referred to as AbNegPA).

10. Standard initial therapy for patients without neurological involvement is 1000 µg intramuscularly ['i.m.'] three times a week for 2 weeks. The BNF advises that patients presenting with neurological symptoms should receive 1000 µg i.m. on alternate days until there is no further improvement.

11. Care must be taken if low dose supplements are prescribed, as such an approach risks the suboptimal treatment of latent and emerging pernicious anaemia with possible inadequate treatment of neurological features.

12. There are arguments against the use of oral cobalamin in initiation of cobalamin therapy in severely deficient individuals who have poor absorption, especially due to pernicious anaemia.

13. Patients with pernicious anaemia need treatment for life regardless of serum cobalamin levels.

Appendix 5

Solicitors briefed about pernicious anaemia

These are the solicitors who have been briefed on how pernicious anaemia can and does have an impact in the workplace:

Northern Ireland

MKB Law (Belfast)
Contact: Tom Johnstone
Tel: 028 9024 2450

Wales

Slater & Gordon
Contact: Rachel Harfield
Tel: 0292 192 1818

England
London

Slater & Gordon
Contact: Mohini Bharania
Tel: 020 7657 1555

Birmingham
Slater & Gordon
Contact: Sarah Evans
Tel: 0121 233 8300

Appendix 6

People of note who have died from pernicious anaemia

At the Pernicious Anaemia Society we are often asked, 'What famous people have, or have had, pernicious anaemia?' This is hard to answer. In the present day people whose diagnosis and treatment are successful generally get on with life without thinking about it, provided they get their injections when they need them; those whose symptoms persist generally abandon their careers and disappear into the background. After considerable searching, the following are some notable people whose lives and work were cut short by pernicious anaemia. If you are aware of others, please bring them to my attention at www.pernicious-anaemia-society.org

Inez Milholland, 6 August 1886 to 25 November 25 1916 – Suffragist, labour lawyer, World War I correspondent and public speaker on women's rights, Milholland died at the age of 30 of pernicious anaemia at a time when no treatment was available.

Annie Oakley, 13 August 1860 to 3 November 1926 – The crackshot sharp-shooter who inspired *Annie Get Your Gun* suffered a decline in health following a serious car accident and she died of pernicious anaemia in 1925 around the time that liver therapy was being developed. She was 66.

Suzanne Lenglen, 24 May 1899 to 4 July 1938 – The early tennis star, who first won Wimbledon women's singles championship in 1919 and was as famous for her daring dress sense as her tennis, suffered from health problems all her life, including asthma as a child. In 1938 she was diagnosed with leukaemia; three weeks later she went blind and then died of pernicious anaemia that same year at the age of just 39.

Alice Marble, 28 September 1913 to 13 December, 1990 – One of the next generation of tennis stars, Alice won five Grand Slam singles finals, starting with the US Championships singles title. At Wimbledon she won the women's singles and doubles, and the mixed doubles. After retiring from tennis she created *Wonder Women of History* for DC Comics but then became a spy for the US during World War II. She eventually died at the age of 77 'weakened by pernicious anaemia'.

Richard O'Connor, 4 August 1851 to 18 November 1912 – This highly successful Australian lawyer and politician, as a representative of New South Wales for the federalist convention was one of the authors of Australia's Federation Act. He died of pernicious anaemia at the age of 61 at a time no treatment was available.

Brigadier Murray William James Bourchier CMG, DSO, VD, MLA, 4 April 1881 to 16 December 1937 – Bourchier was a veteran of the Gallipoli, Egyptian, Sinai, Palestinian and Syrian campaigns in World War I. He subsequently went into politics to fight for the rights of servicemen and became Deputy Premier of Victoria in 1935 and then Victorian Agent General but died from pernicious anaemia and cancer at the age of 56.

J William Billes, 1897 to November 1956 – With his brother, Billes turned the Hamilton Tire and Garage Ltd into the Canadian Tire Corporation Ltd, the most successful Canadian-owned and operated franchise in the country's history that expanded into a nationwide network of dealer-operated associate stores. He died unexpectedly from complications of pernicious anaemia at the age of 59, bequeathing his shares in Canadian Tire to 23 different charitable organisations.

Norman Warne, 1868 to 25 August 1905 – Warne was Beatrix Potter's editor at his family's publishing company, Frederick Warne, where he worked with the author first on *The Tale of Peter Rabbit* (published in 1902) and, when that had proved a bestseller, her other books. As well as their successful working relationship, romance blossomed, despite her parents' opposition, and they were due to be married when Norman died suddenly and unexpectedly of pernicious anaemia at the age of 37.

Sir Laurence Gomme, 18 December 1853 to 23 February 1916 – As founder of the Victoria County History Society and the Folklore Society, Gomme convinced the then London County Council to adopt the 'blue plaque' commemorative scheme in 1901. He was knighted in 1911 but ill health caused him to retire early and he died of pernicious anaemia at the age of 62.

Appendix 7

Ten frequently asked questions

These are the questions the Pernicious Anaemia Society is most frequently asked, together with our answers.

1. What is pernicious anaemia?

Normal people will produce a substance called intrinsic factor in their stomach. The intrinsic factor binds with the vitamin B_{12} from any animal product that has been eaten – fish, dairy meat etc – and transports it to another part of the digestive tract where it enters the bloodstream. People who have pernicious anaemia either do not produce the intrinsic factor or produce antibodies that 'kill off' any intrinsic factor that has been produced. Therefore, people with pernicious anaemia cannot absorb vitamin B_{12} from food and have to have it injected. Vitamin B_{12} is needed to produce healthy red blood cells that transport oxygen around the body.

2. Is it hereditary?

The short answer is yes, but not always. Just because you have it doesn't mean that your children will definitely develop the disease, but there is a tendency for it to run in families.

3. What can I do about it?

You will need to receive supplements of vitamin B$_{12}$ that bypass the absorption problems in your digestive system. Generally that means having injections. You will need these on a regular and life-long basis. With this replacement therapy some patients lead perfectly normal lives just as they did before being diagnosed. Others, for reasons that are not fully understood, still experience the symptoms of the disease even after treatment has begun. This means that some patients will need to develop a 'coping strategy' to best manage their condition, which can mean making small changes to everyday living or having to make substantial changes to the way in which they live and work.

4. Will the symptoms get better, deteriorate or stay the same?

That will depend on the individual. Some patients experience none of the symptoms when they are diagnosed and continue not to feel unwell. Some patients will experience the worst symptoms at diagnosis and see those symptoms disappear once treatment has started. Others, unfortunately, will see no relief from their symptoms once treatment has begun. Your doctor will probably have asked for your ferritin (iron stores) and folate (natural folic acid) to be tested, but if not you might want to suggest that they also are tested as low folate and ferritin can be a cause of symptoms. You shouldn't experience the symptoms getting worse, however, and if this happen, especially if you start to develop neurological symptoms (pins and needles, numbness, and balance problems) you should make an appointment to see your doctor as soon as possible to discuss this with him or her.

5. Can I be cured?

No – as yet there is no cure for pernicious anaemia but you can be treated using replacement therapy B$_{12}$ injections.

6. How is it different from ordinary anaemia?

'Anaemia' means lack of blood or lack of healthy blood. The 'pernicious' in 'pernicious anaemia' means 'fatal'; you cannot transport haemoglobin in your red blood cells. Haemoglobin grabs oxygen and transports it around the body via red blood cells. Without it your cells cannot receive their essential oxygen supply. Because patients with pernicious anaemia cannot absorb vitamin B_{12} they cannot make healthy red blood cells capable of transporting haemoglobin, and thereby oxygen, to where it is needed in the body – which is everywhere. Other types of anaemia include iron-deficiency anaemia – iron is also needed to make haemoglobin – and folate-deficiency anaemia – folate is the natural form of folic acid (vitamin B_9), which again is needed to make healthy blood cells. You can still have pernicious anaemia without being anaemic.

7. I feel my symptoms returning before my injection is due but my doctor refuses to let me have it early. Why?

Most, though not all, doctors believe that, in the UK at least, an injection every three months is adequate, and for some patients it is. There has been no robust research on why some patients need more frequent injections than others, but what is known is that this is the case. You may want to try supplementing your injections by increasing your intake of B_{12} by using sub-lingual tablets or spray, taking 1 mg or 2 mg tablets orally or self-injecting using sub-cutaneous injections of B_{12} from a registered doctor. There are also private clinics that provide injections at a cost. YOU SHOULD DISCUSS ANY OF THESE OPTIONS WITH YOUR DOCTOR BEFORE STARTING SUPPLEMENTATION.

8. Can I overdose on B_{12}?

No; any excess is passed in urine.

9. Am I too young to have pernicious anaemia?

Whatever age you are, you are not too young. Whilst most patients are diagnosed in their 40s, the Pernicious Anaemia Society's youngest member is 12 months old and the oldest is 101. Children and teenagers can develop the condition; it is then known as juvenile pernicious anaemia.

10. I have a deficiency in B$_{12}$ but I have tested negative for intrinsic factor antibodies and parietal cell antibodies – does this mean that I don't have pernicious anaemia?

No – you may still have pernicious anaemia without having the antibodies, as the tests are unreliable.

Glossary

Anaemia: A reduction in the quantity of the oxygen-carrying pigment haemoglobin in the blood. There are over 90 different anaemias. The most common is due to a lack of iron (iron-deficiency anaemia) and is characterised by fatigue, pale skin and (in a blood test) unusually small red blood cells. Pernicious anaemia (see below) is also associated with fatigue and many other symptoms (see page 255) but a blood test may show enlarged red blood cells.

Autoimmune diseases: These are disorders in which the immune system mistakenly attacks the body. The precise cause is unknown but is thought to be associated with ongoing subclinical inflammation. Autoimmune diseases include pernicious anaemia, psoriasis, lupus erythematosus, alopecia and type 1 diabetes.

Blood: Circulating throughout the body, via the arteries and veins, blood is composed of a liquid medium – 'plasma' – and a variety of blood cells (see below) that are suspended in it. Both plasma and red blood cells provide a vehicle for transporting an immense variety of different substances between the various organs and tissues, including oxygen/carbon dioxide (in the red blood cells) and glucose, amino acids, lipids and hormones (in the serum).

B Vitamins: A class of water-soluble vitamins that include:

Vitamin B_1 (thiamine) – discovered in 1910; a good source would be rice bran, plus broccoli, kale, onions

Vitamin B_2 (riboflavin) – discovered in 1920; good sources would be meat, eggs, cheese, almonds

Vitamin B_3 (niacin or nicotinic acid) – discovered in 1936; good sources would be meat, eggs, unrefined grain, peanuts, mushrooms, peas

Vitamin B_5 (pantothenic acid) – discovered in 1931; 'pan' means 'universal reflecting this vitamin is found in many foods

Vitamin B_3 (pyridoxine, pyridoxal, pyridoxamine) – discovered in 1936; good sources would be fish, meat and dairy products, sunflower seeds, pistachio nuts, prunes

Vitamin B_7 (biotin) – discovered in 1931; good sources would be meat (especially organ meats), dairy products and eggs plus green leafy vegetables, green peas, cauliflower

Vitamin B_9 (folate or folic acid) – discovered in 1941; the principal source would be green leafy vegetables

Vitamin B_{12} (various cobalamins – see opposite) – first discovered in 1926; good sources would be organ meats and shell fish; there are very few plant sources of this vitamin.

Blood cell: Also known as blood corpuscles, there are three major categories which each have a specific role. They are all made in the bone marrow:

Red cells (erythrocytes) – these are red because they contain haemoglobin (see below)

White cells (leucocytes) – these are all part of the body's immune system and include the following, which each have a different function:

> granulocytes
> lymphocytes
> monocytes

Platelets – these are small and have no nucleus; they are essential for blood clotting.

Cobalamin: The correct term for vitamin B_{12}. The name refers to the presence of the mineral cobalt at the centre of the vitamin B_{12} molecule. It can exist in several different chemical forms of vitamin B_{12}, depending on variations in part of its chemical structure (the upper axial ligand of the cobalt ion). These forms are:

Cyanocobalamin – the form used in vitamin B_{12} replacement therapy in many countries other than the UK. It is less stable than hydroxocobalamin but much more stable than the so-called active forms.

Hydroxocobalamin – the form used in vitamin B_{12} replacement therapy in the UK. It is more stable than other forms and is thought to last longer in the body, allowing greater time between injections though this is controversial.

Methylcobalamin - an active form of vitamin B_{12}; it relatively unstable, reacting to daylight, but is more stable than adenosylcobalamin.

Adenosylcobalamin – also an active form of vitamin B_{12} and the most unstable.

Enzyme: A protein that, in small amounts, speeds up the rate of a biological reaction without itself being used up in the reaction – in other words, it acts as a catalyst.

Ferritin: An iron-protein complex. It is the main form in which iron is stored in the body, in the liver, spleen and bone marrow.

Fortification (of foods): Also known as 'enrichment', this is the process of adding micronutrients (essential trace elements and vitamins) to food.

Folate: An important B vitamin (vitamin B$_9$). Deficiency, along with deficiency in vitamin B$_{12}$, results in megaloblastic anaemia. Deficiency of folate in the early stages of pregnancy is associated with neural tube defects in the foetus (spina bifida and anencephaly) and there are consequently many advocates of supplementation. However, supplementing folate in the presence of vitamin B$_{12}$ deficiency can mask the presence of pernicious anaemia leading to delayed diagnosis and permanent nerve damage.

Folic acid: A synthetic form of folate (pteroylmonoglutamic acid), used in dietary supplements and food fortification.

Haemoglobin: The major constituent of red blood cells made up of *haem* which contains iron and *globin*, a protein. It is found in the red blood cells and carries oxygen throughout the body to cells for 'aerobic' respiration and carries away carbon dioxide to the lungs.

Intrinsic factor: A glycoprotein secreted in the stomach by the 'parietal cells'. It is essential for the absorption of vitamin B$_{12}$: it binds with the vitamin in the first part of the small intestine (the duodenum) and the B$_{12}$-IF combined substance is then absorbed in the last part of the small intestine (the ileum). Failure to secrete sufficient intrinsic factor leads to a depletion of the vitamin and therefore to pernicious anaemia. On the other hand, the parietal cells may produce sufficient intrinsic factor but the body attack this with intrinsic factory antibody (an autoimmune reaction) and destroy it. The result again is failure to absorb vitamin B_{12} and consequently pernicious anaemia.

Methylation: This is the process whereby cyanocobalamin or hydroxocobalamin is converted into the active form of cobalamin, methylcobalamin.

Nitrous oxide: Also known as 'laughing gas', this is used as an anaesthetic in medicine. It is also used as a recreational drug, causing a sense of euphoria and a dreamlike state. Side effects include fatigue, limb numbness and vitamin B_{12} depletion.

Non-steroidal anti-inflammatory drugs (NSAIDs): These drugs are used to treat pain, rheumatic diseases and inflammatory disorders. They carry a risk of gastro-intestinal side effects which may have an impact on the work of the parietal cells in the stomach.

Parietal cell: These are the cells in the lining of the stomach that produce hydrochloric acid and intrinsic factor; they are also known as oxcyntic cells. They may fail thanks to infection (for instance, from *Helicobacter pylori* in the stomach) or to the body attacking itself (autoimmunity). Intrinsic factor is essential for B_{12} absorption. Hydrochloric acid is essential for breaking down protein in the stomach and allowing vitamin B_{12} to be released from food.

Pernicious anaemia: A form of anaemia resulting from deficiency in vitamin B_{12}. This is because the individual fails to produce the substance (intrinsic factor) that facilitates absorption of B_{12} from the bowel or produces antibodies that destroy any intrinsic factor that has been produced. Pernicious anaemia is characterised by the symptoms listed in Appendix 2 (page 255), resulting from the defective production of red blood cells. The term 'pernicious' reflects the fact that if untreated this form of anaemia is eventually fatal. In severe forms, the nervous system is affected (subacute combined degeneration of the cord secondary to pernicious anaemia – see below). The condition is treated with injections of vitamin B$_{12}$.

Placebo: A 'dummy' medical treatment, prescribed solely for its psychological value. Currently placebos are used in medical trials to judge and compare the benefits of the trial drug as compared with the placebo. When it is thought that the benefits, or lack of benefits, of a treatment are purely psychological (there is no measurable physiological effect) this is called a 'placebo effect'.

Subacute combined degeneration of the cord secondary to pernicious anaemia: This is the term for the neurological disorder complicating a deficiency in vitamin B$_{12}$. The deficiency may be due to lack of B$_{12}$ in the diet (usually only seen in vegans in the developed world) or to malabsorption of vitamin B$_{12}$ in the gut due to low intrinsic factor production, or the production of intrinsic factor antibodies. There is selective damage to the motor and sensory nerve fibres in the spinal cord, resulting in loss of balance and poor limb control. It may also be accompanied by damage to the peripheral nerves and the optic nerve, and by dementia. It is treated by giving vitamin B$_{12}$ injections but this may only halt deterioration; the damage may be irreversible.

Subclinical: This describes a disease that is suspected but is not sufficiently developed to produce definite signs and symptoms in the patient.

Index

absorption/uptake of B_{12}, 25, 105
    problems, 25, **278**
Acheta domesticus, 40
active B_{12} (holotranscobalamin;
    holoTC), 62, 88–92
    tests, 88–92, 219, 221–224
adenosylcobalamin, 22, 225–229, **275**
age and PA, 272
AIRE gene, 115
allergy/allergic reactions, 230–231
    to B_{12}, 155–157
    desensitisation *see* desensitisation
alopecia areata, 118
Alzheimer's disease, 187–188
anaemia, 2, 5–6, **273**
    autoimmune haemolytic, 118
    causes, 6
    defining, 5–6, 271, **273**
    iron-deficiency, 8, 260, 271, 273
    megaloblastic, 87, 161, 184, **276**
    pernicious *see* pernicious
    anaemia

of vitamin B_{12} deficiency, x
Andres (Professor) and Dr Serraj, 35
antibodies (autoimmune)
    intrinsic factor (IFAB), 43,
    84–85, 90, 91, 98, 103, 104,
    109–110, 112, 113, 123, 124, 230,
    232, 262, 272
    parietal cell, 43, 107–109, 119,
    272
    thyroid, 119
anti-epileptic drugs, 19, 50
arthritis
    juvenile idiopathic, 118
    psoriatic, 119
assays *see* diagnosis
atrophic gastric (gastric atrophy),
    42–44, 107
AussieMite, 17
Australia, Marmite versions, 17
autoimmune diseases, 27, **273**
    brain lesions, 167
    co-existing with PA, 117–120

Footnote: The abbreviation PA has been used for pernicious anaemia. Bold
numbers indicate the glossary descriptions and definitions.

279

Footnote: The abbreviation PA has been used for pernicious anaemia. Bold numbers indicate the glossary descriptions and definitions.

Footnote: The abbreviation PA has been used for pernicious anaemia. Bold numbers indicate the glossary descriptions and definitions.

Footnote: The abbreviation PA has been used for pernicious anaemia. Bold numbers indicate the glossary descriptions and definitions.

Footnote: The abbreviation PA has been used for pernicious anaemia. Bold numbers indicate the glossary descriptions and definitions.

Footnote: The abbreviation PA has been used for pernicious anaemia. Bold numbers indicate the glossary descriptions and definitions.

Notes

Diagnosis and Treatment of Chronic Fatigue Syndrome
it's mitochondria, not hypochondria

Dr Sarah Myhill

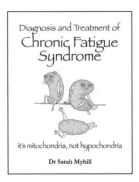

'Dr Myhill has written an extraordinary book. She is the number one authority on CFS in the UK. Whereas many doctors dismiss the condition, she explains what it is, what has gone wrong in the body, using appropriate tests that are not done in mainstream medicine, and tells people what they can do about it. Whereas mainstream medicine only uses drugs to deal with a particular symptom, Dr Myhill explains the reasons why. In my opinion, you will never cure anything unless you understand and deal with the why.'

Dr P J Kingsley

www.hammersmithbooks.co.uk

Sustainable Medicine
whistle-blowing on 21st century medical practice

Dr Sarah Myhill

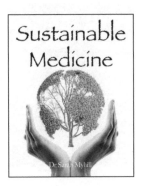

'Dr Myhill addresses the principle causes for the current epidemic of chronic diseases in the Western World and outlines in her unique, no-nonsense way how to explain, prevent, diagnose and successfully treat those conditions for which conventional medicine currently only has an ever increasing amount of potentially dangerous medicines to offer.

This book is an invitation for patients and practitioners alike to move away from a culture of ignorance, restrictive guidelines and blame and to make informed decisions and take responsibility for their own health again.'

Dr Franziska Meuschel MD, PhD, ND, LFhom

www.hammersmithbooks.co.uk

Your Thyroid and How to Keep it Healthy

Dr Barry Durrant-Peatfield

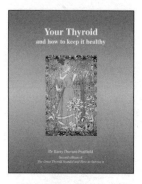

Reprinted 15 times!

Hammersmith Books' all-time best seller continues to be one of the leading books for patients who are struggling with the difficulties of diagnosing and successfully treating underactive thyroid.

Learn how to recognise thyroid dysfunction and its many associated problems and how to take an active part in your own treatment. Learn too about digestive and nutritional issues, including food intolerance and systemic candida infection.

'This book is an absolute must read.'

Positive Health Magazine

www.hammersmithbooks.co.uk